Disclaimer

The contents of this book are provided for informational purposes only and are not intended as a substitute for professional advice or guidance. The author and publisher make no representations or warranties, expressed or implied, regarding the accuracy, completeness, or suitability of the information contained herein for any particular purpose.

Readers are advised to consult with qualified professionals in the relevant field to obtain appropriate advice tailored to their individual circumstances. The author and publisher disclaim any liability, directly or indirectly, for any loss or damage caused or alleged to be caused by the use or reliance upon the information presented in this book.

The inclusion of any external links, references, or resources does not imply endorsement or validation by the author or publisher. These are provided for convenience and additional information, and readers should exercise their own discretion when accessing external content.

This book is a work of fiction or non-fiction (as applicable) and any resemblance to real persons, living or dead, or actual events is purely coincidental. Any opinions expressed within this book are those of the author and do not necessarily reflect the views of the publisher.

The author and publisher reserve the right to make changes to the content, format, or publication schedule of this book without prior notice. This disclaimer is subject to change without notice, and readers are encouraged to review the latest version available.

By reading this book, the reader acknowledges and agrees to the terms of this disclaimer.

First Printing Edition, 2019
Second Printing Edition, 2020
Third Printing Edition, 2021
Fourth Printing Edition, 2022
Fifth Printing Edition, 2023
Sixth Printing Edition, 2024
ISBN 9798873914807

Medical IV Hydratation Therapy Protocols 2024 Update

Doctor Luca Poli

Dedication

This book is dedicated to those whose stories inspired its creation. To the dreamers, whose imagination knows no bounds, and to the resilient spirits that rise after every fall. To the unsung heroes who navigate life's challenges with grace and determination, and to the steadfast friends who stand by our side through every chapter.

In honor of the teachers, mentors, and guides who light the path of knowledge and wisdom, shaping the minds and hearts of future generations. To the seekers of truth, beauty, and meaning, may this work contribute a small spark to the flame of your curiosity.

To the unwavering support of family, whose love provides a foundation for all our endeavors. And to the memory of those who have left indelible imprints on our lives, their legacy forever woven into the fabric of this narrative.

This book is dedicated to the collective human experience—its triumphs, tribulations, and the infinite tapestry of stories that connect us all. May these words resonate with the diverse chords of your own journey and add a melody to the soundtrack of your existence.

CONTENTS

Acknowledgments

I extend my deepest gratitude to those whose support and contributions have been instrumental in bringing this project to fruition.

First and foremost, I want to express my heartfelt appreciation to my family. Your unwavering encouragement, understanding, and love have been the bedrock upon which this endeavor stands. Thank you for being my constant source of inspiration.

To my friends and colleagues, your invaluable insights, discussions, and shared enthusiasm have enriched the narrative in ways I could not have achieved alone. Your camaraderie made the journey all the more enjoyable.

Gratitude is also extended to the readers—those who embark on this literary journey. Your curiosity and engagement with the ideas presented herein are the ultimate reward for any writer.

Finally, I acknowledge the countless writers, thinkers, and creators who have paved the way for the exploration of ideas and the crafting of stories. Your legacy is felt in every page, and I am humbled to contribute to the ongoing conversation.

Thank you to each and every individual who played a part, big or small, in the realization of this project. Your support has been a guiding force, and I am profoundly thankful for your presence on this creative odyssey.

CHAPTER ONE
WHAT IS IV HYDRATATION THERAPY

In the contemporary, fast-paced landscape of today's world, prioritizing optimal health and well-being has become a paramount concern. The prevalence of chronic diseases, heightened stress levels, and inadequate nutrition has prompted a widespread quest for effective strategies to enhance overall health and vitality. Among the emerging solutions, Intravenous (IV) hydration therapy has emerged as a particularly promising avenue, offering individuals the opportunity to replenish essential nutrients, vitamins, and minerals that may be lacking in their daily lives.

The comprehensive guide presented in this book, "Infusion Mastery: The Ultimate Handbook Of Vital Compounds In IV Hydration Therapy" delves into the intricacies of this revolutionary treatment and its potential benefits across a diverse spectrum of conditions. IV hydration therapy involves the administration of vital nutrients, including vitamins, minerals, amino acids, and other essential substances, directly into the bloodstream through intravenous infusion. This method bypasses the digestive system, ensuring a more efficient and effective delivery of crucial components to the body's cells, tissues, and organs, thereby maximizing absorption and utilization of nutrients.

The advantages of IV hydration therapy are multifaceted, extending its utility to a variety of health conditions and bodily symptoms. This book meticulously explores 25 specific conditions and general areas where IV hydration therapy can provide substantial benefits. These encompass a broad range, including fatigue, dehydration, migraines, hangovers, nutrient deficiencies, chronic pain, fibromyalgia, chronic fatigue syndrome, cold and flu symptoms, athletic performance and recovery, jet lag, skin health and anti-aging, detoxification, weight loss, anxiety and stress management, immune system support, asthma and allergies, autoimmune disorders, inflammatory conditions, cognitive function and memory, mood disorders, cancer treatment support, wound healing, anemia, and gastrointestinal disorders.

Throughout the book, a comprehensive examination of the essential components of IV hydration therapy is undertaken, covering vitamins, minerals, amino acids, coenzymes, and other nutrients. By understanding the functions and benefits of each element, readers gain the ability to make informed decisions regarding the most suitable course of action for their unique needs or for those they serve as healthcare professionals.

Detailed discussions on protocols and treatment plans are provided, offering practical guidance on the safe and effective implementation of IV hydration therapy into healthcare regimens. From dosage considerations to administration techniques and contraindications, the book equips readers with the necessary knowledge to optimize their offerings in IV hydration therapy.

"I Infusion Mastery" is indispensable for anyone seeking to enhance health and well-being. Whether you are a healthcare professional, a patient exploring alternative treatments, or simply curious about this innovative approach, the book serves as a valuable resource in the pursuit of optimal health. IV hydration therapy, as detailed in this book, has the transformative potential to address a wide array of health concerns, ultimately contributing to improved overall wellness. Armed with the knowledge gleaned from this resource, readers are empowered to harness the potential of IV hydration therapy and unlock the door to a healthier life, both for themselves and those they aim to serve.

CHAPTER TWO
GUIDELINES FOR UTILIZING THIS BOOK

Over the course of several years, NursePreneurs has successfully implemented its IV Hydration program, centering its approach on the formulation of intravenous solutions. Recognizing a recurring theme in student and customer inquiries, it became evident that there was a substantial interest, if not skepticism, surrounding the specific functionality of each ingredient incorporated into these formulas. While extensive literature exists detailing the chemical composition and molecular arrangements of various substances, the availability of clinically relevant data specifically focused on IV hydration therapy appears to be limited. This dearth of information is compounded by a noticeable lack of comprehensive research interest in this specialized field.

Acknowledging these challenges, we concluded that a dedicated IV hydration clinical handbook should serve as a resource that not only supports the practical aspects of operating an IV hydration clinic but also offers valuable guidance on elucidating the "what and why" of different formula ingredients to layman clients. It is important to recognize that most individuals may not require an in-depth understanding of intricate details such as stereoisomers; rather, their primary concern lies in understanding how a particular ingredient will contribute to their well-being.

It is essential to note that the recommendations provided in this book concerning IV hydration administration quantities and delivery frequencies are rooted in scientific evidence rather than clinical data. Despite conducting an extensive literature search, we have not identified standardized or universally accepted IV hydration formulas. Therefore, it is imperative that the formulas and IV hydration packages employed—whether adapted from peers or uniquely developed—undergo thorough review and approval by a medical director. Furthermore, the development of these formulas should consistently prioritize the best interests of the client.

This book serves as a comprehensive educational resource, offering general insights into IV hydration therapy. It is crucial to emphasize that this publication does not provide patient-specific medical advice and does not replace the guidance or counsel of an individual's qualified medical provider or that of a medical director overseeing a business. As such, any medical decisions or interventions should be made in consultation with appropriately qualified healthcare professionals.

CHAPTER THREE
ESSENTIAL NUTRIENTS

In the ever-evolving landscape of health and well-being, an in-depth comprehension of essential nutrients is vital. This chapter aims to illuminate the nuanced distinctions between vitamins, minerals, and amino acids — crucial elements necessary for the body's optimal functioning.

Vitamins and Minerals: A Comprehensive Overview

Chemical Structure:

Vitamins, organic compounds produced by living organisms, contain carbon. Conversely, minerals are inorganic compounds, naturally occurring and devoid of carbon.

Required Amounts:

Vitamins are classified as fat-soluble (A, D, E, K) or water-soluble (B, C), with the former being stored in the body and the latter requiring regular consumption. Minerals, although needed in small amounts, lack such classification.

Function:

Vitamins contribute to processes such as energy production, immune function, and cell growth. Minerals, on the other hand, play roles in muscle and nerve function, bone health, and the formation of red blood cells.

Sources:

Vitamins are predominantly found in plant and animal-based foods, while minerals originate from soil and water, absorbed by plants and animals. Maintaining adequate levels of both is paramount for good health.

Amino Acids: Foundation of Proteins

Amino acids, the building blocks of proteins, are integral to diverse bodily functions, including muscle growth, immune support, and energy provision. Within IV hydration clinics, amino acids play a pivotal role in replenishing and nourishing the body, especially in cases of dehydration, malnutrition, or conditions affecting protein metabolism.

Exploring Essential Nutrients

Vitamins, minerals, and amino acids stand as indispensable components for various physiological functions. With 13 essential vitamins, each serving a unique purpose, the body relies on this intricate interplay for normal metabolism, growth, and development.

- **Vitamin A:** Vital for vision, immune function, and skin health.

- **Vitamin C:** An antioxidant supporting immune function and collagen synthesis.

- **B Vitamins (B1, B2, B3, B5, B6, B12):** Facilitate energy production, nervous system function, and overall wellness.

- **Minerals:** Inorganic compounds, divided into macrominerals (e.g., calcium, magnesium) and trace minerals (e.g., iron, zinc).

IV Hydration Therapy: Customized Nutrient Delivery

In IV hydration therapy, a targeted approach to nutrient replenishment is embraced, particularly in scenarios where traditional nutrient absorption or metabolism may be compromised. By administering vitamins, minerals, and amino acids directly into the bloodstream, this therapeutic method ensures rapid and efficient absorption, bypassing the digestive system.

The specific nutrients chosen for IV hydration therapy are tailored to individual patient needs and treatment goals. For instance, IV Vitamin C may boost immune function, while a combination of B vitamins enhances energy levels and supports nervous system function. Amino acids like glutamine and arginine aid in post-surgery or illness recovery.

Key Nutrients in IV Hydration Therapy

The selected vitamins, minerals, and amino acids in IV hydration therapy cater to diverse health needs:

- **Vitamin C:** A potent antioxidant fostering immune function and mitigating inflammation.

- **B Vitamins (B1, B2, B3, B5, B6, B12):** Essential for energy production, metabolism, and overall well-being.

- **Magnesium:** Regulates muscle and nerve function, contributing to immune support.

- **Calcium:** Crucial for healthy bones, muscle, and nerve function.

- **Zinc:** Supports the immune system, wound healing, and DNA synthesis.

- **Selenium:** An antioxidant pivotal for immune function and thyroid health.

- **Glutathione:** A potent antioxidant protecting cells and aiding in detoxification.

- **Amino Acids (e.g., arginine, lysine, cysteine):** Fundamental for muscle growth, immune function, and various bodily processes.

Safety Considerations

While IV hydration therapy offers numerous benefits, certain vitamins, minerals, and amino acids must be administered with caution due to potential side effects. For instance, high doses of vitamin A can be toxic, and excessive iron intake may lead to gastrointestinal symptoms. Healthcare providers must carefully evaluate patients' medical histories, ensuring appropriate dosages and nutrient combinations.

This comprehensive exploration serves as an invaluable resource for healthcare professionals, patients seeking alternative treatments, and those intrigued by innovative health approaches. Armed with this knowledge, readers gain a profound understanding of the transformative potential of IV hydration therapy and its role in fostering optimal health and well-being.

CHAPTER FOUR
VITAMINS

In the contemporary realm of healthcare, an intricate understanding of the role of vitamins in various biochemical processes within the human body is imperative. Vitamins, identified as organic compounds, constitute essential micronutrients that the body cannot independently synthesize in adequate quantities and, therefore, necessitate acquisition through dietary sources or supplementation. Their pivotal role in maintaining overall health, fostering growth, and facilitating development cannot be overstated, as they serve as coenzymes, antioxidants, and precursors for indispensable molecules within the body.

The classification of vitamins into two distinct groups, namely fat-soluble and water-soluble, adds complexity to their nuanced role in the intricate balance of bodily functions. Fat-soluble vitamins, including A, D, E, and K, exhibit unique characteristics such as absorption with dietary fats and storage in the liver and adipose tissues. This group's extended half-life in the body makes them susceptible to accumulation, potentially reaching toxic levels if consumed excessively. Vitamin A, essential for vision, immune system function, and tissue maintenance, finds its sources in animal and plant-based foods. Vitamin D, crucial for calcium and phosphorus homeostasis, bone health, and immune function, is synthesized in the skin and present in select foods. Vitamin E acts as an antioxidant, safeguarding cell membranes from oxidative damage, and is prevalent in vegetable oils, nuts, seeds, and leafy greens. Vitamin K, indispensable for blood clotting and bone metabolism, is found in green leafy vegetables, fermented foods, and certain animal products.

On the other hand, water-soluble vitamins, constituting the B complex vitamins and vitamin C, do not accumulate in the body and necessitate regular consumption to maintain optimal levels. The B complex vitamins, encompassing B1 to B12, play integral roles in energy production, brain function, and metabolism. Vitamin C, a potent antioxidant vital for collagen synthesis and immune function, is abundant in fruits and vegetables.

The multifaceted functions of vitamins extend to their participation in various physiological processes within the body. Acting as coenzymes, they assist enzymes in catalyzing essential chemical reactions, with B vitamins being particularly pivotal in metabolic pathways. Additionally, vitamins serve as antioxidants, neutralizing free radicals that could otherwise cause cellular damage. For instance, vitamin C emerges as a robust antioxidant, protecting cells from oxidative stress and contributing to collagen synthesis, crucial for healthy skin, blood vessels, and connective tissues.

The pivotal roles of vitamins extend to hormone synthesis and regulation, immune function, and gene expression. Vitamin D, operating as a hormone, regulates calcium and phosphorus levels, thereby ensuring bone health and preventing conditions such as rickets and osteoporosis. Vitamin A plays a critical role in vision, immune function, and the maintenance of epithelial tissues.

Despite their indispensable nature, inadequate intake of vitamins can lead to deficiencies, manifesting as a spectrum of health problems. Common deficiencies include those of vitamin A, which can lead to night blindness and immune impairment, vitamin D, resulting in conditions like rickets and osteoporosis, and vitamin B12, causing megaloblastic anemia and cognitive dysfunction.

Conversely, excessive intake of certain vitamins can result in toxicities, underscoring the delicate balance required for optimal health. Hypervitaminosis A may lead to symptoms such as nausea, vomiting, and liver damage, while hypervitaminosis D can cause hypercalcemia, kidney stones, and soft tissue calcification.

In striving for balanced vitamin intake, a well-rounded diet comprising a diversity of fruits, vegetables, whole grains, lean proteins, and healthy fats is often sufficient. However, specific populations may be at risk of deficiencies due to age, pregnancy, medical conditions, or dietary restrictions. In such cases, guided vitamin supplementation under healthcare professional oversight becomes imperative to ensure adequate intake.

As we delve further into this chapter, we will provide an in-depth exploration of the vitamins employed in IV Hydration, shedding light on their functions, sources, and potential implications. It's noteworthy that fat-soluble vitamins are generally not utilized in IV therapy due to theoretical risks, including the possibility of a fat embolus. Vitamin D, although included in this list, is typically administered as an intramuscular (IM) shot rather than in an IV bag. Vitamins A, E, and K will not be discussed in the context of IV hydration therapy.

Vitamin C

Vitamin C, scientifically known as ascorbic acid, stands as a pivotal water-soluble vitamin renowned for its robust antioxidant properties. Its multifaceted roles within the human body encompass critical functions, including collagen synthesis, immune system fortification, facilitation of wound healing, enhancement of iron absorption, and robust antioxidant defense against free radicals, thereby mitigating oxidative stress and averting cellular damage.

This comprehensive exploration delves into the nuanced facets of Vitamin C, detailing its indispensable contributions to health and well-being. Central to its significance is collagen production, a protein vital for fortifying connective tissues, skin, bones, and blood vessels. Furthermore, Vitamin C assumes a pivotal role in invigorating the immune system, bolstering immune cell functionality, and fostering antibody production.

Beyond its immune-strengthening capabilities, Vitamin C emerges as a catalyst for efficient wound healing, facilitating tissue repair. Its role extends to augmenting the absorption of non-heme iron from plant-based sources, thereby preventing iron deficiency anemia.

Intriguingly, Vitamin C's antioxidant prowess plays a paramount role in neutralizing harmful free radicals, curbing oxidative stress, and thwarting cellular damage. Given its water-soluble nature, Vitamin C's administration through intravenous infusion presents a mechanism to efficiently deliver these essential components directly into the bloodstream, bypassing the digestive system and optimizing absorption.

Dosage recommendations for Vitamin C intake are delineated based on age, gender, and life stage. The Recommended Dietary Allowance (RDA) spans from 75 mg to 120 mg daily, with additional considerations for smokers.

In the realm of intravenous hydration, the dosage of Vitamin C spans a wide spectrum, ranging from 500 mg to 15,000 mg, contingent upon individual needs and medical conditions. High-dose infusions exceeding 15,000 mg are reserved for specific medical conditions and necessitate vigilant medical supervision.

The applications of Vitamin C infusions are expansive, offering therapeutic support for conditions such as Vitamin C deficiency (scurvy), fatigue, the common cold, iron deficiency anemia, skin aging, oxidative stress-related conditions, and more. High-dose infusions have been explored in the context of cancer treatment support, chronic viral infections, chronic fatigue syndrome (CFS), fibromyalgia, and oxidative stress-related conditions.

However, it is imperative to approach high-dose Vitamin C therapy judiciously, taking into account the patient's medical history, comprehensive blood work, and the specific nuances of each condition. Instances where high-dose Vitamin C may be considered include cancer treatment support, chronic viral infections, chronic fatigue syndrome, and fibromyalgia.

Despite anecdotal reports of enhanced quality of life, improved mood, and increased energy levels among patients, it is crucial to underscore the preliminary nature of such accounts. Rigorous scientific research is indispensable to validate the efficacy and safety of high-dose Vitamin C as a complementary approach in various medical contexts.

The discourse further explores Vitamin C deficiency and toxicity, delineating signs and symptoms associated with both extremes. Contraindications for IV Vitamin C infusions are underscored, encompassing considerations such as a history of kidney stones or kidney disease, hemochromatosis, glucose-6-phosphate dehydrogenase (G6PD) deficiency, and pregnancy or breastfeeding.

The narrative is enriched with insights into the preparation of Vitamin C for IV infusion, storage recommendations, the relatively short half-life of Vitamin C in the body, and considerations regarding its stability. A pertinent section is devoted to the testimonials and experiences of individuals who have undergone high-dose Vitamin C infusions, acknowledging the preliminary nature of anecdotal evidence.

The discourse culminates with a call to promote the benefits of Vitamin C, particularly its role in collagen production, safeguarding skin health, and countering the aging process. IV Vitamin C therapy is presented as an avenue to circumvent absorption barriers associated with oral supplementation, delivering optimal benefits directly into the bloodstream.

Treatment protocols for specific conditions, such as cold and flu, cancer treatment support, chronic fatigue syndrome, and oxidative stress, are provided as educational insights. The comprehensive clinical information section addresses common queries regarding the forms of Vitamin C, daily dosage limits, storage considerations, preparation for IV infusion, and the half-life of Vitamin C in the body.

In essence, this exploration into Vitamin C offers a holistic perspective on its diverse functions, applications in intravenous hydration, and nuanced considerations for optimal healthcare delivery. It serves as a valuable resource for healthcare professionals, patients seeking alternative treatments, and individuals intrigued by the transformative potential of Vitamin C in augmenting overall well-being. As we navigate the intricate landscape of health, this comprehensive guide empowers readers with the knowledge to harness the therapeutic potential of Vitamin C judiciously and efficaciously.

Vitamin B1: Thyamine

Vitamin B1, scientifically known as thiamine, stands as a water-soluble vitamin pivotal to energy metabolism, nerve function, and overall brain health. For nurses embarking on the establishment of an IV hydration clinic, a comprehensive understanding of the benefits, dosage recommendations, treatable conditions, signs of deficiency and toxicity, contraindications, and other pertinent information regarding this indispensable nutrient is imperative.

Benefits of Vitamin B1

Energy Metabolism: Thiamine facilitates the conversion of carbohydrates into energy, thereby supporting cellular function and contributing to overall health.

Nerve Function: Crucial for the proper functioning of the nervous system, thiamine plays a vital role in neurotransmitter production and the maintenance of myelin sheaths.

Brain Health: Thiamine supports cognitive function and memory, and has demonstrated efficacy in treating neurological disorders such as Wernicke-Korsakoff syndrome.

Dosage Recommendations

The Recommended Dietary Allowance (RDA) for thiamine is 1.2 mg/day for adult males and 1.1 mg/day for adult females. In the context of IV hydration, dosages may vary based on formulations and individual needs.

Collaboration with a healthcare professional is essential to determine appropriate dosages for each patient.

Conditions Treated with Vitamin B1

- **Thiamine Deficiency (Beriberi):** Characterized by muscle weakness, peripheral neuropathy, and heart failure, beriberi is effectively treated with thiamine.

- **Wernicke-Korsakoff Syndrome:** This neurological disorder, often associated with chronic alcoholism, causing confusion, memory loss, and ataxia, is addressed with thiamine.

- **Other Neurological Disorders:** Thiamine is incorporated into the treatment plans for conditions like Alzheimer's disease, multiple sclerosis, and peripheral neuropathy.

Signs of Vitamin B1 Deficiency

- Fatigue and weakness

- Muscle wasting and atrophy

- Peripheral neuropathy (tingling, numbness, or pain in extremities)

- Swelling (edema)

- Confusion, memory loss, or cognitive decline

Signs of Vitamin B1 Toxicity

While thiamine toxicity is rare due to efficient excretion, very high doses may lead to adverse effects such as headaches, nausea and vomiting, skin rashes, and hypersensitivity reactions.

Contraindications

Caution is advised in patients with known hypersensitivity to thiamine or any component of the infusion formulation. Additionally, administration should be approached with care in individuals with severe liver or kidney dysfunction.

Special Notes

Beyond treating thiamine deficiency and associated neurological disorders, thiamine has been employed as an adjunct therapy in conditions like diabetic neuropathy, congestive heart failure, and inflammatory bowel disease. Bariatric surgery can induce nutrient deficiencies, including thiamine deficiency, necessitating collaboration with bariatric surgeons to supplement required thiamine stores.

Frequency of Treatments

The frequency of thiamine treatments in an IV hydration setting is contingent on individual patient needs and the specific condition being addressed. Typically, thiamine is administered as part of a vitamin B complex treatment rather than in isolation.

Clinical Information

Forms of Vitamin B1:

Vitamin B1 is available in various forms, including capsules, tablets, injections, and IV infusions.

Daily Dosage Limits:

The recommended daily dosage varies based on age, gender, and health status. For adults, the RDA of vitamin B1 is 1.1-1.2 mg per day, with higher doses recommended for pregnant and lactating women.

Storage of Vitamin B1:

To preserve maximal potency and efficacy, vitamin B1 should be stored in a cool, dry place, away from direct sunlight and heat.

Preparation for IV Infusion:

For IV infusion, vitamin B1 can be prepared by diluting it with sterile water or saline solution. Freshly prepared solutions are crucial to ensure maximal potency and efficacy.

Treatment Protocols:

IV thiamine is employed to treat or prevent thiamine deficiency, which can lead to weakness, fatigue, muscle pain, and neuropathy. Dosage and duration depend on the severity of deficiency and individual response to treatment.

Half-life of Vitamin B1:

The half-life of vitamin B1 in the body is approximately 2 hours, necessitating a continuous supply for sustained levels.

Stability:

Vitamin B1 is relatively stable but can degrade rapidly in the presence of oxygen or in alkaline environments. Proper storage is essential to maintain potency.

In conclusion, this detailed exploration of Vitamin B1 serves as a comprehensive guide for nurses entering the realm of IV hydration therapy, ensuring a thorough understanding of its intricacies and applications in healthcare settings.

Vitamin B2: Riboflavin

Vitamin B2, scientifically known as riboflavin, stands as a pivotal water-soluble vitamin, contributing significantly to crucial physiological functions such as energy production, cellular growth, and the preservation of skin and eye health. This essential nutrient plays a fundamental role in the formation of flavin coenzymes (FAD and FMN), integral in metabolic processes involving the conversion of carbohydrates, fats, and proteins into energy. Additionally, riboflavin supports cellular growth, reproduction, and the body's antioxidant defenses, thereby ensuring the maintenance of optimal cellular function.

Riboflavin's impact extends to the realms of skin, hair, and nail health, while also exerting positive effects on vision and protecting the eyes from oxidative stress. Understanding the benefits, recommended dosage, conditions treated, signs of deficiency and toxicity, contraindications, and other pertinent information is imperative for those seeking to optimize health through riboflavin supplementation.

The Recommended Dietary Allowance (RDA) for riboflavin is established at 1.3 mg/day for adult males and 1.1 mg/day for adult females. However, in an Intravenous (IV) hydration setting, dosages may vary depending on specific formulations and individual needs, emphasizing the necessity of consultation with a healthcare professional to determine appropriate dosages tailored to each patient.

Conditions treated with Vitamin B2 range from addressing riboflavin deficiency (ariboflavinosis) to mitigating the frequency and severity of migraines and treating specific eye disorders, such as cataracts and corneal disorders. Signs of riboflavin deficiency include cracked and red lips (cheilosis), inflammation and soreness of the mouth and tongue (stomatitis and glossitis), scaly, greasy skin rashes (seborrheic dermatitis), anemia, sensitivity to light (photophobia), and eye fatigue.

Notably, riboflavin toxicity is rare, with excess amounts efficiently excreted through urine. While there are no known toxic effects associated with high riboflavin intake from food or supplements, extremely high doses may cause harmless bright yellow-orange urine discoloration.

In an IV hydration setting, there are no known contraindications for riboflavin supplementation. However, caution is advised for patients with a known hypersensitivity to riboflavin or any component of the infusion formulation.

Riboflavin's role extends beyond addressing deficiency and migraines, as it may serve as an adjunct therapy for conditions like anemia, enhancing iron absorption, and mitigating oxidative stress related to various health conditions.

The frequency of riboflavin treatments in an IV hydration setting is contingent on individual patient needs and the specific condition being treated, typically forming part of a vitamin B Complex treatment rather than administered in isolation.

Clinical information pertaining to riboflavin includes its availability in various forms (capsules, tablets, and liquids), the recommended daily dosage limits, proper storage conditions to maintain potency, preparation for IV infusion, treatment protocols, half-life, stability, and factors affecting its degradation.

By delving into the depths of this comprehensive understanding of Vitamin B2, individuals, healthcare professionals, and those curious about optimizing health can make informed decisions, harnessing the potential of riboflavin to promote overall well-being.

Vitamin B3: Niacin

Vitamin B3, commonly known as niacin, is a water-soluble vitamin that assumes a pivotal role in various physiological processes, including energy metabolism, cellular function, and the maintenance of skin, nerve, and digestive health. Its benefits extend across several dimensions:

Energy Metabolism: Niacin is a crucial component in the formation of nicotinamide adenine dinucleotide (NAD) and its phosphate form (NADP), acting as essential coenzymes in metabolic processes. These processes include the conversion of carbohydrates, fats, and proteins into energy.

Cellular Function: Niacin supports cellular growth, reproduction, and DNA repair, contributing to the overall health of tissues and organs.

Skin, Nerve, and Digestive Health: Niacin is indispensable for maintaining healthy skin, supporting proper nerve function, and ensuring the smooth operation of the digestive system.

Dosage Recommendations:

The Recommended Dietary Allowance (RDA) for niacin stands at 16 mg/day for adult males and 14 mg/day for adult females, expressed as niacin equivalents (NE). In an IV hydration setting, niacin doses may vary based on the specific formulation and individual needs. Consulting with a healthcare professional is imperative to determine the appropriate dosage for each patient.

Conditions Treated with Vitamin B3:

Niacin is employed in treating various conditions, including niacin deficiency (pellagra), hyperlipidemia, and migraines.

Signs of Vitamin B3 Deficiency:

Dermatitis, diarrhea, and dementia are indicative of niacin deficiency. Dermatitis may manifest as skin rashes, particularly in sun-exposed areas, accompanied by a characteristic "necklace" rash around the neck.

Signs of Vitamin B3 Toxicity:

High doses of niacin can lead to toxicity, causing adverse effects such as flushing, gastrointestinal symptoms (nausea, vomiting, and diarrhea), liver damage, and impaired glucose tolerance.

Contraindications:

Caution is advised in individuals with a known hypersensitivity to niacin or any component of the infusion formulation. Patients with liver disease, diabetes, peptic ulcers, or gout should also approach niacin use cautiously due to the potential exacerbation of these conditions.

Special Notes - Specific Conditions Treated with Niacin:

Beyond treating niacin deficiency and hyperlipidemia, niacin has been explored as an adjunct therapy for osteoarthritis and age-related macular degeneration (AMD).

Frequency of Treatments:

The frequency of niacin treatments in an IV hydration setting is individualized based on the patient's needs and the specific condition being addressed. Typically, niacin is part of a vitamin B complex or NAD treatment and is not administered in isolation.

Clinical Information:

A thorough exploration of clinical information includes the forms of vitamin B3 (niacinamide, nicotinic acid), daily dosage limits, storage considerations, preparation for IV infusion, treatment protocols, half-life, stability, and the potential therapeutic benefits in various health conditions.

This detailed discussion provides a comprehensive understanding of vitamin B3, ensuring that healthcare professionals and individuals alike are well-informed about its diverse functions, applications, and considerations in both oral and intravenous forms.

Vitamin B5: Pantothenic Acid

Vitamin B5, also scientifically referred to as pantothenic acid, stands as a water-soluble vitamin, assuming a pivotal role in diverse physiological processes, notably energy metabolism, cellular function, and the synthesis of essential compounds integral to proper bodily functioning. The multifaceted benefits of Vitamin B5 encompass pivotal contributions to energy metabolism, as it constitutes a fundamental component of coenzyme A, essential for the breakdown of carbohydrates, fats, and proteins to generate energy. Furthermore, Vitamin B5 plays a crucial role in cellular processes such as DNA and RNA production, as well as the synthesis of cellular membranes. Notably, its involvement in the production of coenzyme A and the synthesis of fatty acids positions Vitamin B5 as vital for maintaining healthy skin and hair.

In terms of recommended daily intake, the Recommended Dietary Allowance (RDA) for pantothenic acid is established at 5 mg/day for both adult males and females. However, in the context of IV hydration therapy, dosages may vary contingent on specific formulations and individual requirements. Hence, it is imperative to seek consultation with a healthcare professional to determine the most appropriate dosage for each patient.

Vitamin B5 is employed in treating various conditions, including pantothenic acid deficiency, which can manifest as symptoms like fatigue, insomnia, and gastrointestinal disturbances. Additionally, Vitamin B5 has demonstrated efficacy in addressing acne by reducing sebum production and plays a crucial role in wound healing and tissue repair.

Identification of Vitamin B5 deficiency is essential, and signs may include fatigue, insomnia, gastrointestinal disturbances, and numbness and tingling in the extremities. It is noteworthy that Vitamin B5 toxicity is a rare occurrence, as high doses are generally well-tolerated. However, excessive intake may result in side effects such as diarrhea and stomach upset, emphasizing the importance of using Vitamin B5 supplements under the guidance of a healthcare professional, particularly considering potential interactions with certain medications.

Pantothenic acid should be approached with caution in individuals with known hypersensitivity to the vitamin or any component of the infusion formulation. Furthermore, patients with kidney disease should exercise caution, as high doses of pantothenic acid may exacerbate renal function.

The alcohol derivative of pantothenic acid, known as dexpanthenol, finds application in IV hydration therapy for wound healing and skin and hair health. Dexpanthenol stimulates cell proliferation and migration while reducing inflammation, making it valuable in promoting skin and tissue healing. The frequency of Vitamin B5 treatments in an IV hydration setting is contingent on individual patient needs and the specific condition being addressed, often incorporated into a comprehensive vitamin B complex.

This comprehensive exploration of Vitamin B5 extends to its various forms, including capsules, tablets, and liquid supplements, as well as its natural occurrence in foods like meat, poultry, fish, whole grains, and legumes. Storage guidelines recommend a cool, dry environment away from direct sunlight and heat for Vitamin B5 supplements.

Preparing Vitamin B5 for IV infusion involves dissolving it in sterile water or saline solution, with the resultant solution either used immediately or refrigerated for later administration. While Vitamin B5 exhibits a relatively short half-life of approximately 2-3 hours in the body, it remains a stable compound unaffected by heat, light, or air.

In the realm of treatment protocols, Vitamin B5 has been subject to research for its potential therapeutic benefits across diverse health conditions, encompassing acne, wound healing, and stress. Nevertheless, establishing optimal dosages and durations for supplementation necessitates further exploration, with variations likely depending on individual responses and health conditions. For instance, protocols for acne treatment might involve daily doses of 2-10 grams of pantothenic acid over 12 weeks, while wound healing protocols may encompass daily doses of 2-3 grams over a period of up to 4 weeks.

In conclusion, the information encapsulated in this extensive discourse on Vitamin B5 is essential for healthcare professionals, patients exploring alternative treatments, and individuals keen on understanding the potential benefits and applications of IV hydration therapy. As a dynamic element in health and wellness, Vitamin B5 possesses the capacity to influence a myriad of health concerns, contributing significantly to the pursuit of optimal health. Armed with the insights gleaned from this discourse, readers are empowered to navigate the complexities of Vitamin B5 and IV hydration therapy, ultimately steering toward a healthier and more informed life.

Vitamin B6: Pyridoxine

Vitamin B6, scientifically known as pyridoxine, stands as a vital water-soluble nutrient, playing a pivotal role in numerous physiological functions such as metabolism, neurotransmitter synthesis, and immune function. For nursing professionals aspiring to establish an IV hydration clinic, a comprehensive understanding of this essential nutrient becomes imperative. This involves delving into its benefits, dosage recommendations, conditions treated, signs of deficiency and toxicity, contraindications, and other pertinent information.

Benefits of Vitamin B6

1. **Metabolism:** Vitamin B6 actively participates in amino acid metabolism, the foundational process for protein building, facilitating the conversion of food into energy.

2. **Neurotransmitter synthesis:** Crucial for the synthesis of neurotransmitters like serotonin and dopamine, Vitamin B6 contributes to mood regulation.

3. **Immune function:** It plays a role in the production of white blood cells, vital components for immune function.

Dosage Recommendations

The recommended dietary allowance (RDA) for vitamin B6 ranges from 1.3 to 1.7 mg/day for adult men and women. In an IV hydration context, dosages may vary based on formulations and individual needs, necessitating consultation with a healthcare professional to determine optimal patient-specific dosages.

Conditions Treated with Vitamin B6

1. **Nausea and vomiting:** Frequently used to address nausea and vomiting linked to pregnancy, chemotherapy, or other medical conditions.

2. **Neurological conditions:** Applied in the treatment of neurological issues like seizures, migraines, and neuropathy.

3. **Anemia:** Involved in the synthesis of hemoglobin, the protein in red blood cells responsible for oxygen transport.

Signs of Vitamin B6 Deficiency

- Anemia

- Depression

- Dermatitis

- Neurological symptoms such as seizures and neuropathy

Signs of Vitamin B6 Toxicity

Excessive intake can lead to sensory neuropathy, ataxia, and skin lesions. However, toxicity is rare and typically occurs with undue supplementation.

Contraindications

Caution is advised in individuals with known hypersensitivity to vitamin B6 or components of the infusion formulation. Additionally, patients with kidney disease should be treated cautiously due to potential exacerbation of renal function.

Special Notes - What Specific Conditions Does Pyridoxine Treat?

Pyridoxine has been employed to treat diverse conditions, including nausea and vomiting associated with pregnancy or chemotherapy, neurological conditions such as seizures, migraines, and neuropathy, and anemia.

Frequency of Treatments

Treatment frequency depends on individual needs and the specific condition being addressed, with vitamin B6 commonly part of a vitamin B Complex.

Clinical Information

1. **Forms of Vitamin B6:** Available in capsules, tablets, liquid supplements, and naturally occurring in foods such as poultry, fish, whole grains, vegetables, and nuts.

2. **Daily Dosage Limits:** Vary based on individual needs, with a general recommended daily intake of 1.3-1.7 milligrams for adults.

3. **Storage:** Supplements should be stored in a cool, dry place, away from direct sunlight and heat.

4. **Preparation for IV Infusion:** Dissolved in sterile water or saline solution, the solution should be used immediately or refrigerated for later use.

5. **Treatment Protocols:** Studies explore potential therapeutic benefits for various health conditions, with dosage and duration varying based on individual needs and response to treatment.

6. **Half-life:** Approximately 20-30 hours in the body.

7. **Stability:** A relatively stable compound unaffected by heat, light, or air.

This detailed exploration underscores the importance of Vitamin B6 in healthcare, emphasizing the need for informed decision-making by healthcare professionals considering IV hydration therapy.

Vitamin B7: Biotin

Vitamin B7, more commonly known as biotin, is a water-soluble vitamin crucial for various physiological functions, particularly the metabolism of carbohydrates, fats, and proteins. This essential nutrient plays a pivotal role in maintaining overall health, with notable benefits spanning metabolic processes, the promotion of healthy skin, hair, and nails, and potential assistance in blood sugar control, particularly in individuals with diabetes.

Benefits of Vitamin B7:

1. **Metabolism:** Biotin is a key player in the metabolism of carbohydrates, fats, and proteins.

2. **Healthy Skin, Hair, and Nails:** Biotin contributes to the maintenance of healthy skin, hair, and nails.

3. **Blood Sugar Control:** Biotin exhibits potential in improving blood sugar control, particularly beneficial for individuals with diabetes.

Dosage Recommendations:

The recommended daily intake of biotin for adults is 30 mcg. However, in an IV hydration setting, dosages may vary based on specific formulations and individual needs. It is imperative to consult with a healthcare professional to determine the appropriate dosage for each patient.

Conditions Treated with Vitamin B7:

1. **Skin Conditions:** Biotin may be utilized to address various skin conditions such as dermatitis and eczema.

2. **Hair and Nail Health:** Biotin may enhance the strength and quality of hair and nails.

3. **Blood Sugar Control:** Biotin may aid in improving blood sugar control in individuals with diabetes.

Signs of Vitamin B7 Deficiency:

1. Skin rash or dermatitis

2. Brittle nails

3. Hair loss

4. Neurological symptoms, such as depression and lethargy

Signs of Vitamin B7 Toxicity:

Biotin toxicity is rare, with no established toxicity level identified. However, high doses may cause side effects such as skin rash and gastrointestinal disturbances, and interactions with certain medications may occur.

Contraindications:

While generally safe, individuals with known hypersensitivity to biotin or components of the infusion formulation should avoid supplementation.

Special Notes - Specific Conditions Treated by Biotin:

Biotin has been applied to treat conditions including skin disorders (dermatitis, eczema), hair and nail health, and blood sugar control in individuals with diabetes.

Frequency of Treatments:

The frequency of vitamin B7 treatments in an IV hydration setting depends on individual patient needs and the specific condition being treated. Typically, vitamin B7 is part of a vitamin B Complex infusion.

Clinical Information:

1. **Forms of Vitamin B7:** Available in various forms, including capsules, tablets, and liquid supplements. Naturally found in foods like egg yolks, liver, nuts, and whole grains.

2. **Daily Dosage Limits:** Daily dosage varies, with a generally recommended intake of 30 micrograms for adults. Higher doses may be used for specific medical conditions.

3. **Storage:** Supplements should be stored in a cool, dry place, away from direct sunlight and heat.

4. **Preparation for IV Infusion:** Prepared by dissolving in sterile water or saline solution, the solution should be used immediately or refrigerated.

5. **Treatment Protocols:** Studies on potential therapeutic benefits in hair loss, diabetes, and skin disorders exist, with optimal dosage and duration varying based on individual needs and responses.

6. **Half-Life:** Vitamin B7 has a short half-life of approximately 2 hours.

7. **Stability:** A stable compound unaffected by heat, light, or air.

This detailed exploration provides a comprehensive understanding of vitamin B7, ensuring informed decisions and effective utilization of its potential benefits in various health contexts.

Vitamin B9: Folic Acid

Vitamin B9, known as folic acid or folate, represents a crucial water-soluble vitamin essential for various physiological functions, prominently including DNA production and red blood cell formation. This vital nutrient plays a pivotal role in fostering health and is particularly recognized for its involvement in fundamental processes such as red blood cell production, DNA production and repair, and the development of the fetal neural tube during pregnancy.

Benefits of Vitamin B9:

1. **Red Blood Cell Production:** Folic acid is intricately involved in the production of red blood cells, which play a vital role in oxygen transport throughout the body.

2. **DNA Production:** Folic acid is indispensable for the synthesis and repair of DNA.

3. **Neural Tube Development:** Critical for the development of the fetal neural tube during pregnancy.

Dosage Recommendations:

The recommended daily intake for adults is 400 mcg of folic acid. In an IV hydration setting, dosages may fluctuate based on formulation specifics and individual needs. A healthcare professional's consultation is imperative to ascertain the appropriate dosage for each patient.

Conditions Treated with Folic Acid:

1. **Anemia:** Folic acid is employed in the treatment of anemia resulting from a deficiency in red blood cells.

2. **Pregnancy:** Essential for fetal neural tube development, reducing the risk of certain birth defects.

3. **Cardiovascular Disease:** May contribute to lowering the risk of cardiovascular disease by reducing homocysteine levels in the blood.

Signs of Vitamin B9 Deficiency:

- Anemia

- Fatigue

- Neural tube defects in infants born to mothers with a deficiency

- Diarrhea

Signs of Vitamin B9 Toxicity:

While folic acid toxicity is rare, high doses may mask vitamin B12 deficiency symptoms, potentially leading to neurological damage. Additionally, high doses can induce gastrointestinal symptoms and interact with certain medications.

Contraindications:

Folic acid is generally safe; however, individuals hypersensitive to the vitamin or infusion components should avoid supplementation.

Special Notes - What Specific Conditions Does Folic Acid Treat?

Folic acid is utilized to treat and prevent conditions such as anemia, neural tube defects during pregnancy, and for the reduction of heart and cardiovascular disease risk.

Frequency of Treatments:

The frequency of vitamin B9 treatments in an IV hydration setting varies based on individual needs and the specific condition being addressed.

Clinical Information:

1. **Forms:** Vitamin B9 is available in various forms, including capsules, tablets, and liquid supplements.

2. **Dosage Limits:** Daily dosage may vary but generally recommended at 400 micrograms for adults.

3. **Storage:** Supplements should be stored in a cool, dry place away from sunlight and heat.

4. **Preparation for IV Infusion:** Dissolved in sterile water or saline solution, the solution should be used immediately or refrigerated.

5. **Treatment Protocols:** Studies explore potential therapeutic benefits in conditions such as anemia, neural tube defects, and cardiovascular disease. Optimal dosage and duration depend on individual response to treatment.

Additional Information:

- **Half-life:** Approximately 3 hours in the body.

- **Stability:** Relatively stable, unaffected by heat, light, or air.

This detailed exploration of Vitamin B9 serves as a comprehensive resource for healthcare professionals, patients seeking alternative treatments, or anyone interested in the nuanced complexities of leveraging folic acid for health optimization.

Vitamin B12: Cobalamin

Vitamin B12, scientifically known as cobalamin, represents a water-soluble vitamin that plays a pivotal role in numerous physiological functions, encompassing DNA production, the formation of red blood cells, and the maintenance of nerve function. For nursing professionals aspiring to establish an IV hydration clinic, a comprehensive understanding of vitamin B12 is imperative. This encompasses knowledge about its benefits, recommended dosages, treated conditions, signs of deficiency and toxicity, contraindications, and other pertinent information concerning this essential nutrient.

Benefits of Vitamin B12:

1. **Red Blood Cell Production:** Vitamin B12 is indispensable for the synthesis of red blood cells, crucial for oxygen transport throughout the body.

2. **Nerve Function:** Critical for the proper functioning of the nervous system.

3. **DNA Production:** Involved in the production and repair of DNA.

Dosage Recommendations:

The recommended daily intake for adults is 2.4 micrograms. However, in an IV hydration setting, dosages may vary based on formulation and individual needs, necessitating consultation with a healthcare professional for personalized assessment.

Conditions Treated with Vitamin B12:

1. **Anemia:** Used to treat anemia resulting from red blood cell deficiency.

2. **Nerve Damage:** Deficiency can lead to nerve damage, and supplementation may alleviate symptoms.

3. **Cognitive Decline:** May help slow cognitive decline in age-related memory loss.

Signs of Vitamin B12 Deficiency:

1. Anemia

2. Fatigue

3. Neurological symptoms like tingling or numbness in extremities

4. Cognitive decline

Signs of Vitamin B12 Toxicity:

Rare; no established toxicity level identified.

Contraindications:

Generally safe, but those hypersensitive to vitamin B12 or infusion components should avoid supplementation.

Special Notes:

Different forms of B12 include hydroxocobalamin, methylcobalamin, cyanocobalamin, and adenosylcobalamin. Methylcobalamin, preferred in IV hydration, is considered more bioavailable and effective.

Frequency of Treatments:

Varies based on individual needs and the condition treated. IM shots may be administered weekly, and for weight loss, lipoB12 injections are generally given.

Clinical Information:

1. **Forms of Vitamin B12:** Tablets, capsules, injections, and naturally found in animal products.

2. **Daily Dosage Limits:** Recommended daily intake is 2.4 micrograms for adults.

3. **Storage:** Keep B12 supplements in a cool, dry place, away from sunlight and heat.

4. **Preparation for IV Infusion:** Dissolve in sterile water or saline solution, use immediately, or refrigerate.

5. **Treatment Protocols:** Varied for conditions like pernicious anemia; optimal dosage and duration not universally established.

6. **Half-Life:** Approximately 6 days.

7. **Stability:** Stable in food, but vulnerable in supplement form; store in optimal conditions to preserve potency.

In conclusion, this intricate understanding of Vitamin B12 is essential for healthcare professionals, patients exploring alternative treatments, or anyone intrigued by this innovative approach. The transformative potential of IV hydration therapy, with a focus on Vitamin B12, can contribute significantly to overall health and wellness. Armed with this knowledge, individuals are empowered to harness the potential of Vitamin B12 and optimize their well-being.

Vitamin D: Cholecalciferol (D3) and Ergocalciferol (D2)

Vitamin D, a crucial fat-soluble vitamin, plays an integral role in numerous bodily functions, ranging from bone health and immune function to the regulation of calcium and phosphorus levels. While Intravenous (IV) hydration therapy typically focuses on water-soluble vitamins like B vitamins, there are instances where vitamin D supplementation through IV infusion becomes necessary. However, it's essential to note that Vitamin D is most commonly administered through Intramuscular (IM) injection.

The benefits of Vitamin D are manifold, impacting bone health by facilitating the absorption and metabolism of calcium and phosphorus, crucial for maintaining optimal bone health. It also plays a pivotal role in modulating the immune system, with deficiency linked to an increased risk of infections and autoimmune diseases. Additionally, Vitamin D may contribute to mood regulation and the prevention of depression.

Dosage recommendations for vitamin D vary, with a daily intake of 600-800 IU recommended for adults. Higher doses may be necessary based on specific conditions or risk factors. In an IV hydration setting, dosages may differ depending on the formulation and individual needs.

This book addresses various conditions that can benefit from Vitamin D supplementation, including Vitamin D deficiency, osteoporosis, autoimmune diseases, and more. Recognizing signs of deficiency, such as muscle weakness, bone pain or loss, fatigue, and an increased risk of infections, is crucial.

While Vitamin D toxicity is rare, it can occur with excessively high doses, leading to symptoms like nausea, vomiting, and kidney damage. Contraindications include individuals with hypercalcemia or a history of kidney stones, who should avoid high-dose vitamin D supplementation. Consultation with a healthcare professional is imperative to determine appropriate dosage and potential contraindications for each patient.

Importantly, Vitamin D is not typically administered through IV infusion due to its fat-soluble nature, which can lead to accumulation in the body's fat stores, posing a risk of toxicity. Monitoring vitamin D levels through blood tests is essential to ensure proper supplementation. Optimal vitamin D levels vary, with most experts recommending a blood level of at least 30 ng/mL for optimal health, and potentially higher levels for enhanced bone health and immune function.

The book provides insights into the different forms of vitamin D, D2 (ergocalciferol) and D3 (cholecalciferol), their origins, and potential variations in effectiveness. It also delves into treatment protocols for various medical conditions, offering guidelines on dosage, duration, and administration.

Frequently asked questions about vitamin D, including its forms, daily dosage limits, storage, and stability, are addressed in a comprehensive manner. The half-life of vitamin D, approximately 2-3 weeks, is discussed, emphasizing factors influencing its variability.

Ultimately, this resource is indispensable for healthcare professionals, patients seeking alternative treatments, or those intrigued by the innovative approach of IV hydration therapy with Vitamin D. It provides a thorough understanding of the intricacies of Vitamin D supplementation, equipping readers with the knowledge to optimize health and well-being effectively.

CHAPTER FIVE
MINERALS

Minerals, as indispensable inorganic substances, intricately contribute to a myriad of physiological processes within the human body, playing pivotal roles in sustaining overall health. Their significance lies in the promotion of robust bone and teeth structure, facilitation of nerve impulse transmission, regulation of fluid balance, and support for optimal muscle function. The array of minerals essential for human well-being encompasses calcium, iron, magnesium, phosphorus, potassium, sodium, chloride, zinc, copper, manganese, selenium, iodine, chromium, and molybdenum. Each mineral serves a unique function critical to the intricate balance of bodily processes.

Distinguishing themselves from organic compounds like vitamins, which the body requires in minute quantities for health maintenance and deficiency prevention, minerals are inorganic and cannot be synthesized internally. Instead, they must be acquired through dietary sources or supplementation. Vitamins are further classified as either water-soluble (e.g., vitamin C and B vitamins) or fat-soluble (e.g., vitamins A, D, E, and K), while minerals fall into major and trace mineral categories based on their quantity requirements. Major minerals, such as calcium and magnesium, are necessitated in larger quantities, while trace minerals, including zinc and selenium, are essential in smaller amounts.

Both minerals and vitamins function as essential nutrients vital for maintaining good health and preventing disease. While Intravenous (IV) therapy stands out as an efficient method for the swift and direct replenishment of minerals, there are certain considerations to bear in mind:

1. **Electrolyte Imbalances:** Some minerals, like sodium, potassium, and magnesium, function as electrolytes crucial for fluid balance, nerve function, and muscle activity. Imbalances in these minerals may lead to issues such as muscle cramps, irregular heartbeats, and seizures.

2. **Kidney Function:** The kidneys play a pivotal role in filtering and eliminating excess minerals from the body. If kidney function is compromised, the administration of high doses of minerals through IV therapy may result in mineral buildup and toxicity.

3. **Allergic Reactions:** Certain individuals may exhibit allergies or sensitivities to specific minerals, potentially causing reactions such as hives, swelling, and breathing difficulties.

4. **Infection:** Like any medical procedure involving needle insertion, there is a risk of infection associated with IV therapy. Strict adherence to sterile techniques is crucial during the administration of IV therapy.

5. **Overdose:** Excessive doses of minerals administered through IV therapy can lead to toxicity and adverse effects, underscoring the importance of careful dosage considerations.

Commonly included minerals in IV hydration formulations, such as magnesium, calcium, zinc, copper, selenium, and chromium, are integral for sustaining cellular function and energy production. Their incorporation into IV hydration therapy serves as a means for individuals to optimize their health and well-being. In the subsequent section, we will delve into the specific benefits, recommended dosages, and potential side effects associated with each of these minerals, providing a comprehensive understanding of their role in IV hydration therapy.

Magnesium

Magnesium is an indispensable mineral that plays a pivotal role in numerous physiological processes within the human body. Its involvement in energy production, muscle and nerve function, as well as the regulation of blood pressure and glucose levels underscores its significance in maintaining optimal health. Beyond these fundamental functions, magnesium has proven benefits for bone and heart health, and it has been associated with alleviating symptoms of migraine headaches and enhancing sleep quality.

Dosage recommendations for magnesium intake are contingent upon factors such as age and sex. The standard daily intake for adults ranges between 310 and 420 mg/day. However, for those receiving magnesium through intravenous (IV) therapy, the dosage is tailored to the specific condition being treated and the severity of the deficiency.

Magnesium is widely employed in IV hydration therapy to address various conditions, including hypomagnesemia (low magnesium levels), arrhythmias, asthma, migraines, and preeclampsia in pregnant women. Additionally, it is utilized to enhance athletic performance, reduce muscle soreness, and manage chronic pain.

Symptoms of magnesium deficiency encompass muscle cramps, weakness, fatigue, irritability, and abnormal heart rhythms. Severe deficiency can manifest as seizures, changes in personality, and numbness or tingling in the extremities. Conversely, magnesium toxicity is rare but may occur with excessive administration, leading to symptoms such as nausea, vomiting, low blood pressure, and difficulty breathing, with severe cases potentially resulting in cardiac arrest.

Certain contraindications exist, and individuals with renal impairment or severe cardiac disease are advised to avoid high doses of magnesium. Ideal candidates for magnesium infusion therapy include those experiencing symptoms of magnesium deficiency, pregnant women with preeclampsia, and individuals with conditions like asthma or migraines.

Magnesium is often administered in conjunction with other minerals, such as calcium, or combined with amino acids like taurine and arginine to optimize athletic performance and reduce muscle soreness.

The frequency of magnesium infusion therapy varies based on the specific condition and the severity of the deficiency. Treatment is typically administered over several hours and may be repeated as needed.

Magnesium is available in different forms, including magnesium oxide, magnesium citrate, magnesium chloride, and magnesium glycinate. It is also present in various food sources such as leafy green vegetables, nuts, and whole grains.

Storage guidelines for magnesium supplements emphasize keeping them in a cool, dry place, shielded from direct sunlight and heat, to maintain maximal potency and efficacy. For IV infusion, magnesium can be prepared by reconstituting it with sterile water or saline solution, with freshly prepared solutions ensuring optimal potency.

The therapeutic potential of magnesium in conditions like hypertension, migraines, and constipation has been studied, but optimal dosage and duration of supplementation remain areas of ongoing research, with protocols varying based on individual needs and treatment response. The half-life of magnesium depends on the dose and administration route, with intravenous magnesium having a relatively short half-life of approximately 1 to 2 hours, while orally administered magnesium has a longer half-life of around 30 hours. Magnesium is a stable compound unaffected by heat or light, and it is highly soluble in water, requiring proper storage to preserve its efficacy.

Calcium

Calcium, an essential mineral, plays a pivotal role in various bodily functions, encompassing the formation and upkeep of healthy bones and teeth, nerve function, muscle contraction, and blood clotting. This comprehensive exploration underscores the criticality of calcium in maintaining the body's overall mineral balance and its involvement in diverse cellular and biochemical processes.

The administration of calcium via intravenous (IV) hydration therapy necessitates careful consideration of factors such as age, weight, medical history, and the specific condition being addressed. Dosages typically range between 500 to 1500 mg per day, with a maximum dosage capped at 2000 mg per day. The versatility of IV calcium extends to treating an array of medical conditions, including hypocalcemia, osteoporosis, muscle cramps, tetany, and specific arrhythmias. Furthermore, it finds application in addressing acute hyperkalemia, signifying its broad therapeutic potential.

The manifestation of signs indicating calcium deficiency, such as muscle weakness, cramps, brittle bones, and neurological symptoms, underscores the vital role of maintaining adequate calcium levels. Conversely, excessive calcium intake may lead to toxicity, resulting in symptoms like nausea, vomiting, abdominal pain, constipation, and kidney stones, with severe cases potentially culminating in cardiac arrest.

Calcium infusion, however, is not without considerations. Contraindications include individuals with hypercalcemia or a history of kidney stones, necessitating cautious use in those with heart disease, hypertension, or a history of blood clots. Ideal candidates for calcium infusion comprise individuals unable to take oral supplements, those with severe calcium deficiency, and those with medical conditions requiring higher calcium levels than achievable through diet alone.

This exploration extends to the coadministration of calcium with other minerals and electrolytes in IV hydration therapy, offering a nuanced understanding of treatment protocols, including dosages, administration techniques, contraindications, and precautions.

The book further provides a deep dive into clinical information, addressing various forms of calcium, daily dosage limits, storage considerations, and the preparation of calcium for IV infusion. It sheds light on treatment protocols, elucidating the potential therapeutic benefits of calcium in health conditions such as osteoporosis, hypertension, and hypocalcemia. The varying half-lives of calcium, depending on the route of administration, are explored, with stability considerations emphasizing the need for proper storage to maintain maximal potency and efficacy.

In essence, this comprehensive guide serves as an invaluable resource for healthcare professionals, patients seeking alternative treatments, and those intrigued by the intricacies of IV hydration therapy. The transformative potential of calcium, when harnessed with knowledge from this book, presents an opportunity to enhance health and well-being across a myriad of conditions.

Zinc

Zinc, an indispensable mineral, plays a pivotal role in a multitude of physiological functions within the human body. Its involvement in cell growth, immune function, DNA synthesis, wound healing, and various metabolic processes underscores its significance. Beyond these fundamental roles, zinc boasts antioxidant properties, safeguarding cells against oxidative stress, and actively participates in the regulation of insulin secretion and glucose metabolism. Furthermore, zinc is instrumental in maintaining the health of the skin, hair, and nails.

Dosage recommendations for zinc are rooted in the recommended dietary allowance (RDA), set at 8-11 mg per day for adult men and women, respectively, with a safe upper limit of 40 mg per day for adults. However, in the context of IV therapy, the dosage may fluctuate based on an individual's health condition and the therapeutic intent.

Zinc emerges as a versatile tool in treating various health conditions, including zinc deficiency, diarrhea, Wilson's disease, acne, and symptoms associated with cold and flu. The repercussions of zinc deficiency are extensive, spanning growth retardation, compromised immune function, and delayed wound healing. Conversely, excessive zinc intake can lead to toxicity, marked by symptoms such as nausea, vomiting, abdominal cramps, diarrhea, and headaches. Prolonged exposure to high zinc levels may result in copper deficiency, anemia, and weakened immune function.

In determining candidates for zinc infusion, individuals with severe zinc deficiency or malabsorption issues are identified as potential beneficiaries. Zinc infusion finds utility in treating conditions like diarrhea, Wilson's disease, and symptoms associated with cold and flu. The integration of zinc with other minerals and amino acids in IV therapy can enhance therapeutic outcomes.

The frequency of zinc infusion varies depending on the individual's health condition and the intended purpose of the therapy, with healthcare provider recommendations guiding the frequency and duration of the treatment. Noteworthy is the use of zinc in addressing cold and flu symptoms owing to its immune-boosting properties. Zinc gluconate is the preferred form for IV therapy, known for its ready availability and good bioavailability. Conversely, zinc carbonate is deemed unsuitable for IV therapy due to its potential to induce a rapid drop in blood pressure and a higher risk of adverse effects.

Clinical information surrounding zinc encompasses its various forms, daily dosage limits, storage considerations, preparation for IV infusion, treatment protocols, and the half-life of zinc. While zinc is a stable compound unaffected by heat or light, proper storage in a cool, dry place away from direct sunlight and heat is crucial to ensure maximal potency and efficacy. The book further explores the therapeutic benefits of zinc in conditions like the common cold, wound healing, and age-related macular degeneration, elucidating that optimal dosage and duration may vary based on individual responses to treatment. Understanding the pharmacokinetics of zinc, including its half-life, is vital for informed decision-making in clinical settings.

Copper

Copper, an essential mineral with pivotal roles in various physiological processes, stands as a cornerstone in the human body. Its involvement in critical functions such as red blood cell production, immune system maintenance, and energy production underscores its significance. This comprehensive exploration into the realm of copper sheds light on its myriad benefits, serving as a key component in enzymes pivotal for cellular functions, including antioxidant defense, iron metabolism, and connective tissue synthesis.

Understanding the nuances of copper intake is imperative, with the recommended daily intake for adults set at 900 micrograms. However, the dosage for copper infusion is contingent upon individual health status and the specific medical condition being addressed. The versatile applications of copper in medical treatments extend to conditions such as anemia, osteoporosis, and copper deficiency. Moreover, the anti-inflammatory and antioxidant properties of copper offer potential benefits in managing conditions like arthritis, cardiovascular disease, and certain neurological disorders.

Exploring the spectrum of copper's impact, the book delves into the signs of both deficiency and toxicity. Copper deficiency can manifest in symptoms ranging from anemia to impaired immune function, while excess copper intake may lead to nausea, vomiting, abdominal pain, and, in severe cases, liver and kidney damage. Acute copper poisoning is rare but can result from ingesting large amounts of copper-containing substances, while chronic toxicity may stem from prolonged exposure to elevated copper levels.

Contraindications for copper infusion are outlined, emphasizing caution for individuals with Wilson's disease or liver disease, who may experience altered copper metabolism. Ideal candidates for copper infusion include those with copper deficiency, anemia, or medical conditions warranting copper supplementation.

The intricate interplay of copper with other compounds in IV therapy is explored, offering insights into its potential coadministration with amino acids, vitamins, and minerals based on individual health conditions. The frequency of copper infusion is tailored to the specific medical condition and overall health status of the individual.

In addition to these considerations, the book provides valuable clinical information on copper, covering its various forms, daily dosage limits, storage requirements, preparation for IV infusion, and treatment protocols. A blood test for monitoring copper levels is emphasized to prevent potential adverse effects during infusion therapy.

This comprehensive guide serves as an invaluable resource for healthcare professionals, patients seeking alternative treatments, and those intrigued by the intricate role of copper in optimizing health. The transformative potential of copper, when harnessed with knowledge from this book, becomes a powerful tool for enhancing well-being across diverse medical conditions.

Selenium

Selenium, an essential mineral, occupies a pivotal role in various physiological functions, encompassing antioxidant activity, thyroid hormone metabolism, and immune system function. This comprehensive exploration of selenium, as detailed in the book, delves into its multifaceted benefits, acting as a cofactor for enzymes and proteins vital for cellular function and homeostasis. Beyond its fundamental role, selenium is implicated in preventing specific cancers and cardiovascular diseases.

In the realm of IV hydration therapy, the appropriate dosage of selenium is contingent on individual needs and health conditions. The recommended dietary allowance (RDA) for adults stands at 55 micrograms (mcg) per day, with an upper limit of 400 mcg per day. The book underscores the importance of consulting a healthcare provider before initiating supplementation.

Selenium deficiency can lead to diverse health issues, including muscle weakness, fatigue, impaired immune function, and an elevated risk of certain cancers. IV selenium therapy emerges as a potential solution for individuals at risk of deficiency or those with conditions benefiting from increased selenium levels.

Signs of selenium deficiency, as outlined, encompass cognitive decline and, in severe cases, Keshan disease—a heart condition linked to selenium-poor soils. While selenium toxicity is rare, excessive supplementation can lead to nausea, vomiting, hair loss, and, in extreme cases, severe respiratory and cardiovascular complications.

The book provides crucial information on contraindications, cautioning against selenium supplementation for individuals with allergies, those taking specific medications, pregnant women, and children. It sheds light on ideal candidates for selenium infusion, including individuals with deficiencies or specific health conditions such as thyroid disorders, cardiovascular disease, and cancer.

Exploring selenium's synergy with other compounds, the book discusses its potential combination with antioxidants like vitamin C and E, as well as minerals like zinc, to support immune function. The frequency of selenium IV therapy, tailored to individual needs, is outlined, emphasizing the importance of adhering to healthcare provider recommendations.

Special notes highlight the significance of blood tests for measuring selenium levels and the variations in absorption rates and bioavailability of different selenium forms. Sodium selenite emerges as the most commonly used form of selenium in IV therapy.

The clinical information section provides a comprehensive overview, addressing the forms of selenium, daily dosage limits, storage considerations, preparation for IV infusion, and treatment protocols. Selenium's therapeutic potential in conditions like thyroid disease, cancer, and cardiovascular disease is acknowledged, with the caveat that optimal dosage and duration vary based on individual responses.

The half-life of selenium is elucidated, varying with the form and individual metabolism. While selenium is relatively stable, it is sensitive to oxidative damage, necessitating proper storage away from heat and light to maintain potency and efficacy. The book provides a thorough understanding of selenium, offering valuable insights for healthcare professionals, patients, and those interested in innovative health approaches.

Chromium

Chromium, an indispensable mineral, assumes a pivotal role in the intricate metabolism of carbohydrates, lipids, and proteins within the human body. Its significance is particularly emphasized in the proper functioning of insulin, a hormone crucial for regulating blood sugar levels. Beyond its fundamental role in insulin function, chromium has demonstrated potential benefits in weight management, glucose metabolism, and cardiovascular health.

The recommended daily intake of chromium for adults is set between 20-35 micrograms per day, a range that ensures optimal physiological functions. However, in the realm of IV hydration therapy, dosages may be subject to individualized treatment plans and patient-specific needs. Consulting with a healthcare provider becomes paramount in determining the precise dosage suitable for IV administration.

Chromium supplementation holds promise in addressing various medical conditions associated with blood sugar regulation, such as insulin resistance, type 2 diabetes, and metabolic syndrome. Additionally, its potential impacts on weight loss, athletic performance, and cognitive function are subjects of ongoing scientific exploration.

The absence of adequate chromium levels may manifest in signs such as impaired glucose tolerance, insulin resistance, elevated blood sugar levels, fatigue, irritability, and weight gain. On the contrary, excessive chromium intake can lead to toxicity, resulting in adverse effects such as gastrointestinal issues, skin reactions, and damage to vital organs, including the liver and kidneys. While severe cases of chromium poisoning are rare and typically associated with industrial accidents or environmental contamination, the potential for harm underscores the importance of adhering to recommended dosage levels.

Contraindications for chromium supplementation include individuals with liver or kidney disease, those taking specific medications like antacids or corticosteroids, and pregnant individuals. Determining the suitability for chromium infusion involves careful consideration of specific medical conditions and potential deficiencies, necessitating consultation with a healthcare provider.

Chromium may be combined with other nutrients and compounds, such as B vitamins and amino acids, in IV administration, contingent on the specifics of the treatment plan. The frequency of IV administration varies based on individual needs and the treatment plan, requiring close collaboration with a healthcare provider.

Notably, the measurement of chromium levels in the body is not routinely conducted due to the absence of a widely accepted method for assessing chromium status. However, individuals with specific medical conditions or known chromium deficiencies may benefit from testing to determine their chromium levels.

The clinical information section elucidates the various forms of chromium available, daily dosage limits, storage considerations, preparation for IV infusion, treatment protocols, and the compound's half-life. This comprehensive guide serves as a valuable resource for healthcare professionals and individuals alike, navigating the intricate landscape of chromium supplementation, its potential therapeutic benefits, and the nuanced considerations surrounding its usage in IV hydration therapy.

Summary

The integral role of minerals in upholding the holistic health and well-being of the human body necessitates their thoughtful incorporation into the realm of IV hydration therapy. Within this context, the delicate equilibrium of essential elements such as calcium, magnesium, zinc, chromium, copper, and selenium emerges as a pivotal consideration, exerting a profound influence on an individual's recovery trajectory, overall performance, and general health outcomes.

Recognizing the nuanced impact of each mineral is paramount, as their collective contribution extends beyond mere supplementation, profoundly influencing cellular and physiological processes. The intricate interplay between these minerals underscores the need for a judicious approach in administering them through IV hydration therapy, ensuring their therapeutic benefits while averting the potential risks of toxicity or imbalances.

Healthcare professionals undertaking the administration of minerals in IV hydration therapy must navigate the intricate terrain of individual patient needs. Tailoring treatments to the unique requirements of each patient involves a meticulous evaluation of their medical history, existing health conditions, and specific mineral deficiencies. This personalized approach demands astute clinical judgment to ascertain the optimal dosage, thereby mitigating potential side effects and complications.

The judicious integration of minerals into IV hydration therapy holds the promise of not only addressing existing deficiencies but also fostering enhanced recovery and bolstering overall health. Through a nuanced understanding of the distinctive roles and significance attributed to each mineral, healthcare practitioners can craft bespoke IV hydration treatments that resonate with the specific health goals and challenges faced by their patients.

In conclusion, the strategic incorporation of minerals into IV hydration therapy emerges as a dynamic and essential facet of modern healthcare. By upholding the principles of precision and individualization, healthcare professionals can harness the therapeutic potential of minerals to augment recovery, fortify performance, and propel patients toward a state of optimal health and well-being.

CHAPTER SIX
AMINO ACIDS

Amino acids, as fundamental constituents of proteins, play a pivotal role in the growth and repair of tissues within the human body. With a repertoire of 20 different types, amino acids can be categorized as essential or nonessential. Essential amino acids, vital for bodily functions, cannot be synthesized internally and necessitate dietary intake or supplementation. Conversely, nonessential amino acids are produced by the body, although certain circumstances, such as illness, injury, or intense exercise, may warrant supplementation.

The book meticulously details the nine essential amino acids, each contributing uniquely to physiological processes such as muscle growth and repair, immune function, and energy production. Histidine, isoleucine, leucine, lysine, methionine, phenylalanine, threonine, tryptophan, and valine each fulfill distinctive roles in maintaining optimal health.

In contrast, the 11 nonessential amino acids can be synthesized within the body. However, under specific conditions, such as illness or intense physical activity, the body's production may fall short, prompting the need for supplementation. Alanine, arginine, asparagine, aspartic acid, cysteine, glutamic acid, glutamine, glycine, proline, serine, and tyrosine contribute to various physiological functions, from glucose metabolism and energy production to immune support and wound healing.

While essential amino acids take precedence in IV hydration therapy formulas due to their indispensable nature, small amounts of certain nonessential amino acids, such as glycine, may be included for their role in collagen synthesis and wound healing. Alanine, another nonessential amino acid, may be added to promote healthy blood sugar levels.

The book broadens its scope to encompass amino acid derivatives, including glutathione, taurine, carnitine, citrulline, ornithine, and N-acetylcysteine (NAC). These compounds, structurally related to amino acids, undergo modifications that impart unique functionalities. For instance, glutathione, derived from cysteine, glutamic acid, and glycine, acts as a powerful antioxidant. Taurine, while structurally similar to amino acids, lacks a carboxyl group and is found in various tissues, contributing to the regulation of electrolytes, neurotransmitter modulation, and cell membrane stability. Carnitine, synthesized from lysine and methionine, facilitates the transport of fatty acids for energy production.

The inclusion of ornithine in the urea cycle, citrulline in ammonia removal and nitric oxide production, and NAC as a precursor to glutathione highlights the diverse roles of amino acid derivatives. These compounds, meticulously explored in the book, contribute significantly to various metabolic processes and health outcomes.

In conclusion, the intricate exploration of amino acids, their essential and nonessential classifications, and their derivatives in IV hydration therapy constitutes a valuable resource for healthcare professionals and individuals seeking to optimize health and well-being. The nuanced understanding of these fundamental elements offers insights into personalized treatment strategies, emphasizing the potential benefits of amino acid supplementation in diverse physiological contexts.

Derivative amino acids

The decision to opt for amino acid derivatives over the actual amino acids in supplementation is influenced by several considerations, each grounded in the pursuit of enhanced bioavailability, specific health benefits, and lower toxicity. Amino acid derivatives may exhibit increased bioavailability, making them more readily absorbed and utilized by the body than their parent amino acids. This heightened bioavailability can stem from differences in molecular structure, solubility, or other factors affecting metabolic processes.

One compelling reason to choose amino acid derivatives lies in the potential for specific health benefits that may not be inherent in the original amino acid. For instance, taurine, a derivative of cysteine and methionine, showcases antioxidant properties and may contribute to the regulation of blood pressure, thereby supporting healthy heart function.

In certain instances, amino acid derivatives may offer a more favorable safety profile with lower toxicity and fewer side effects compared to their parent amino acids. An illustrative example is N-acetylcysteine (NAC), an oral supplement derived from cysteine, commonly employed to bolster liver function and promote respiratory health. Notably, NAC is recognized for its safety and tolerance even at higher doses, reinforcing its appeal in supplementation.

The decision to supplement with amino acid derivatives or actual amino acids is contingent upon various factors, including an individual's health status, dietary intake, and specific health objectives. This chapter focuses on amino acids and their derivatives deemed practical for intravenous (IV) hydration, emphasizing those commonly utilized in this context.

Among the essential amino acids frequently employed in IV hydration, histidine is recognized for potential anti-inflammatory and antioxidant effects. Leucine is often included for its purported benefits in muscle building and repair, while lysine may find its place for immune-boosting effects. Methionine, known for potential detoxifying effects, and threonine, which may support immune function, are also commonly used. Tryptophan, with its potential mood-boosting effects, and valine, contributing to muscle-building and repair, complete the roster of essential amino acids in IV hydration.

Nonessential amino acids integral to IV hydration include alanine, promoting healthy blood sugar levels; arginine, beneficial for circulation and cardiovascular issues; glutamine, involved in energy production, muscle recovery, and immune regulation; and glycine, contributing to collagen synthesis and wound healing.

In the realm of amino acid derivatives in IV hydration, key players include glutathione, recognized for its antioxidant properties; taurine, known for its role in blood pressure regulation; carnitine, contributing to energy metabolism; ornithine, playing a role in ammonia detoxification; citrulline, involved in nitric oxide production; and NAC, already mentioned for its liver support and respiratory health benefits.

In essence, the strategic selection between amino acid derivatives and their source amino acids in IV hydration depends on a nuanced evaluation of individual health profiles, dietary considerations, and specific wellness goals. This chapter serves as an in-depth exploration of these considerations, providing valuable insights into the practical applications of amino acids and their derivatives in the context of intravenous hydration therapy.

Exploring the Significance of Essential Amino Acids

Histidine

Histidine, classified as a semi-essential amino acid, assumes a pivotal role in diverse physiological processes within the human body. Although not commonly utilized as the primary component in intravenous (IV) hydration solutions, histidine can be incorporated into these solutions to offer supplementary nutritional support in specific scenarios.

The multifaceted benefits of histidine encompass its involvement in physiological processes, such as histamine production—a compound integral to immune response and inflammation. Histidine also contributes to pH balance regulation, participates in red and white blood cell production, and may possess antioxidant properties, thereby aiding in wound healing.

Determining the appropriate dosage of histidine for IV infusion relies on individual patient needs and therapy goals, with typical dosages ranging from 2-4 grams per day for adults. It is crucial to exercise caution, as excessive doses of histidine may lead to toxicity.

Histidine finds application in IV solutions designed for patients facing malnutrition or conditions affecting nutrient absorption. Although histidine deficiency is rare, patients with certain genetic disorders may exhibit symptoms like anemia, poor wound healing, and fatigue. Conversely, histidine toxicity resulting from excessive doses may manifest as headaches, nausea, and vomiting.

Caution is advised when administering histidine to patients with liver or kidney disease, as these organs are responsible for amino acid metabolism. Additionally, patients with a history of allergies or asthma should use histidine cautiously, as it may exacerbate these conditions.

Ideal candidates for histidine infusion include malnourished individuals, those with compromised nutrient absorption, and patients recovering from injury or surgery. Histidine may be combined with other compounds and amino acids in IV hydration solutions to enhance nutritional support.

The frequency of histidine infusion is contingent on patient-specific needs and therapy goals, with dosages typically ranging from 2-4 grams per day for adults. The infusion frequency may vary, administered daily or several times per week based on individual requirements.

Histidine, besides its use in IV hydration solutions, may also serve as a natural flavor enhancer in certain food products, owing to its slightly sweet and savory taste.

Clinical information regarding histidine includes details about its forms, daily dosage limits, storage instructions, preparation for IV infusion, and treatment protocols. Histidine supplements, available in various forms like capsules, tablets, powders, and liquids, should be stored in a cool, dry place away from direct sunlight and heat.

Histidine's therapeutic benefits have been explored in conditions such as rheumatoid arthritis and anemia. Treatment protocols may involve daily doses of 2 grams for rheumatoid arthritis and 15-25 milligrams per kilogram of body weight for anemia, each for specific durations.

Histidine, characterized by a relatively short half-life of 2-3 hours, remains stable under conditions of heat, light, and air. However, proper storage is essential to maintain maximal potency and efficacy.

Leucine

Leucine, classified as an essential amino acid, assumes a pivotal role in protein synthesis and muscle maintenance. While not typically utilized as the primary constituent in IV hydration solutions, leucine can be incorporated into these solutions to provide supplementary nutritional support in specific scenarios. This comprehensive exploration of leucine encompasses its benefits, dosage recommendations, conditions it may address, signs of deficiency and toxicity, contraindications, suitable candidates for leucine infusion, potential combinations with other compounds or amino acids, frequency of treatments, and pertinent clinical information.

Leucine, a branched-chain amino acid (BCAA), demonstrates involvement in protein synthesis and muscle maintenance. Scientific evidence indicates that leucine promotes muscle protein synthesis, enhancing muscle growth and aiding recovery post-exercise. Additionally, leucine exhibits potential anti-inflammatory properties and may contribute to improved insulin sensitivity, offering advantages for individuals with type 2 diabetes.

The recommended dosage of leucine for IV infusion hinges on patient-specific needs and therapeutic goals, typically ranging from 4-8 grams per day for adults. However, caution is warranted, as excessive doses of leucine may lead to toxicity.

Although leucine is not frequently employed as a standalone therapy, its addition to IV hydration solutions can provide nutritional support, especially for patients facing malnutrition or difficulties in nutrient absorption. Signs of leucine deficiency, albeit rare, encompass muscle weakness, fatigue, and impaired wound healing, while toxicity symptoms include nausea, vomiting, and diarrhea.

Contraindications stipulate cautious use in individuals with liver or kidney disease, and those allergic to peanuts or soy, given their leucine content. Potential candidates for leucine infusion include malnourished individuals, those with compromised nutrient absorption, and athletes seeking to enhance muscle growth and recovery.

Leucine may be combined with other compounds and amino acids in IV hydration solutions, particularly with other BCAAs like isoleucine and valine, amplifying nutritional and athletic performance support. The frequency of leucine infusion is contingent upon patient needs, with typical dosages administered daily or several times per week.

Clinical information surrounding leucine encompasses its various forms, daily dosage limits, storage guidelines, preparation for IV infusion, and treatment protocols. Leucine, obtained from protein-rich foods or available as supplements in diverse forms, including capsules, tablets, powders, and liquids, should be stored in a cool, dry place away from direct sunlight and heat. The half-life of leucine is relatively short— approximately 1-2 hours—and it is considered a stable compound unaffected by heat, light, or air. However, to ensure maximal potency and efficacy, proper storage practices are recommended.

In conclusion, this detailed exploration of leucine offers a comprehensive understanding of its potential benefits and applications in IV hydration therapy, providing valuable insights for healthcare professionals, patients, and those interested in optimizing nutritional support for various health conditions.

Lysine

Lysine, an essential amino acid, occupies a pivotal role in protein synthesis and immune function within the human body. While not commonly employed as the primary component in Intravenous (IV) hydration solutions, lysine can be strategically added to such solutions to provide supplemental nutritional support in specific scenarios.

The multifaceted benefits of lysine encompass its involvement in critical physiological processes such as enzyme and hormone production, collagen and protein formation, and the regulation of immune function. Additionally, lysine exhibits potential antiviral properties, contributing to the reduction in severity and duration of cold sores caused by the herpes simplex virus.

Dosage recommendations for lysine in IV infusion are contingent upon individual patient needs and therapeutic goals. Typically, dosages range from 2 to 4 grams per day for adults, with a caveat on avoiding excessive doses to prevent toxicity.

While lysine is not commonly employed as a standalone therapy for any specific medical condition, it finds application in IV hydration solutions as an additional nutritional component. For instance, lysine may be incorporated into IV solutions for malnourished patients or those with conditions affecting nutrient absorption.

Lysine deficiency is rare, given its essential role in bodily functions; however, in specific cases, such as certain genetic disorders, symptoms may include fatigue, anemia, and decreased appetite. Conversely, excessive doses of lysine can lead to toxicity, resulting in symptoms like nausea, vomiting, and diarrhea.

Caution is advised in administering lysine to patients with liver or kidney disease, as these organs are responsible for amino acid metabolism. Furthermore, individuals allergic to lysine or with a history of kidney stones should use lysine cautiously.

Good candidates for lysine infusion include malnourished individuals, those with conditions affecting nutrient absorption, or those with compromised immune systems recovering from injury or surgery. Lysine infusion may also be combined with other compounds and amino acids in IV therapy to enhance nutritional support.

The frequency of lysine infusion is contingent upon patient-specific needs and therapeutic objectives. Usual dosages range from 2 to 4 grams per day for adults, with the infusion administered daily or several times per week, tailored to individual requirements.

The clinical information section provides insights into various aspects of lysine, including its forms, daily dosage limits, storage requirements, preparation for IV infusion, treatment protocols, and its half-life. Lysine's stability, being relatively unaffected by heat, light, or air, underscores the importance of proper storage to ensure maximal potency and efficacy.

This comprehensive guide serves as a valuable resource for healthcare professionals and individuals seeking in-depth knowledge on lysine and its potential therapeutic applications in IV hydration therapy.

Methionine

Methionine, an essential amino acid, assumes a pivotal role in various physiological processes such as protein synthesis, detoxification, and the formation of critical molecules like glutathione. While not typically the primary component in IV hydration solutions, methionine can be incorporated into these solutions to offer supplementary nutritional support in specific scenarios.

The multifaceted benefits of methionine extend to its involvement in protein and DNA synthesis, gene expression regulation, and its critical role in the production of glutathione—an essential antioxidant and detoxifying molecule. The amino acid may also possess anti-inflammatory properties and contribute to improved liver function.

Dosage recommendations for methionine in IV infusion hinge upon individual patient needs and therapeutic goals, typically ranging from 1 to 2 grams per day for adults. It is crucial to exercise caution as excessive doses may lead to toxicity.

While not frequently employed as a standalone therapy, methionine finds application in IV hydration solutions to provide nutritional support in circumstances such as malnourishment or conditions affecting nutrient absorption. Signs of methionine deficiency, though rare, may include fatigue, muscle weakness, and decreased immunity. Conversely, excessive doses may result in toxicity, presenting symptoms like nausea, vomiting, and diarrhea.

Contraindications for methionine use involve caution in patients with liver or kidney disease, a history of peptic ulcer disease, or those taking certain medications. Individuals with sulfur allergies may require special consideration, although methionine, containing sulfur in the form of sulfhydryl groups, is not typically associated with sulfur allergies.

Potential candidates for methionine infusion include malnourished individuals, those with conditions affecting nutrient absorption, or patients with liver-related concerns or recovering from injury or surgery. Methionine may be combined with other compounds and amino acids in IV therapy to enhance its nutritional support.

The frequency of methionine infusion is individualized based on patient needs, typically ranging from 1 to 2 grams per day for adults, administered daily or several times per week.

Special considerations highlight methionine's sensitivity to light, prompting the need for storage in a cool, dry, and dark place to prevent degradation. IV methionine solutions should be stored in light-resistant containers or covered with light-proof wraps during administration to maintain potency and efficacy.

Clinical information underscores the various forms of methionine, including supplements available in capsules, tablets, powders, and liquid forms. Storage instructions, preparation for IV infusion, treatment protocols, and half-life considerations further contribute to the comprehensive understanding of methionine's role in healthcare.

Studies on methionine's therapeutic benefits across conditions like liver disease, depression, and cancer underscore its potential, but optimal dosages and durations remain subjects of ongoing research, subject to individual responses and needs. Methionine's short half-life of approximately 3-4 hours underscores the need for careful consideration under conditions of high oxidative stress or toxin exposure. Although stable against heat, its susceptibility to light necessitates meticulous storage practices.

Threonine

Threonine, classified as an essential amino acid, assumes a pivotal role in vital physiological processes, including protein synthesis and immune function. Although not commonly employed as the primary component in intravenous (IV) hydration solutions, threonine may be introduced to these solutions to furnish supplementary nutritional support in specific contexts. The multifaceted benefits of threonine encompass its involvement in the production of enzymes and hormones, the formation of collagen and other proteins, and the regulation of immune function. Additionally, threonine may contribute positively to gut health and digestive improvement.

In the context of IV infusion therapy, the appropriate dosage of threonine is contingent upon the individual patient's needs and the therapeutic goals, typically ranging from 1 to 2 grams per day for adults. It is imperative to note that excessive threonine doses may pose toxicity risks.

While threonine is not typically employed as a standalone therapy for specific medical conditions, it can be incorporated into IV hydration solutions to provide additional nutritional support. For instance, threonine may be included in IV solutions for malnourished patients or those with conditions affecting nutrient absorption from food.

Threonine deficiency is a rare occurrence given its essential nature for proper bodily function. However, in specific instances, such as patients with certain genetic disorders or those on severely restricted diets, threonine deficiency may manifest with symptoms like fatigue, irritability, and decreased immunity. Conversely, excessive threonine doses may lead to toxicity symptoms such as nausea, vomiting, and diarrhea.

Caution is warranted in patients with liver or kidney disease, as these organs are responsible for metabolizing amino acids. Threonine should also be used cautiously in individuals allergic to threonine or with a history of kidney stones.

Potential candidates for threonine infusion include malnourished individuals, those with conditions affecting nutrient absorption, or patients with compromised immune systems, injuries, or post-surgery recovery. Threonine may be combined with other compounds and amino acids in IV hydration solutions, enhancing its therapeutic effects.

The frequency of threonine infusion hinges on the patient's specific needs and therapeutic goals, with typical dosages ranging from 1 to 2 grams per day for adults. Infusion may be administered daily or several times per week, aligning with the patient's requirements.

Clinical information on threonine covers its various forms, daily dosage limits, storage recommendations, preparation for IV infusion, and treatment protocols. Threonine supplements, found in protein-rich foods and available in various forms, including capsules, tablets, powders, and liquid forms, should be stored in a cool, dry place away from direct sunlight and heat. The short half-life of threonine, approximately 2-3 hours, necessitates careful consideration under conditions of high oxidative stress or toxin exposure. Threonine is generally stable, resilient to heat, light, and air, but prudent storage practices are essential to ensure optimal potency and efficacy.

Threonine has been subject to studies exploring its potential therapeutic benefits in diverse health conditions, such as wound healing, liver disease, and intestinal disorders. However, optimal dosage and duration of threonine supplementation for different health conditions remain subjects of ongoing research, contingent upon individual responses and needs. The comprehensive coverage of threonine in this professional discourse positions it as a valuable resource for healthcare professionals, researchers, and individuals seeking a nuanced understanding of its applications in IV hydration therapy.

Tryptophan

Tryptophan, an essential amino acid, assumes a pivotal role in the synthesis of key molecules such as serotonin and melatonin, contributing to mood regulation and sleep. While not typically employed as the primary component in intravenous (IV) hydration solutions, tryptophan can be added to such solutions to offer supplementary nutritional support in specific scenarios.

The manifold benefits of tryptophan encompass its involvement in the production of serotonin and melatonin, impacting mood regulation, sleep, immune function, and digestion. Dosage recommendations for IV infusion hinge on patient-specific needs and therapeutic objectives, typically ranging from 1-2 grams per day for adults. It is crucial to exercise caution, as excessive doses of tryptophan may result in toxicity.

Although not commonly used as a standalone therapy, tryptophan may be incorporated into IV hydration solutions to provide additional nutritional support. This may be particularly beneficial for patients who are malnourished or experiencing challenges in nutrient absorption due to certain medical conditions.

Tryptophan deficiency is a rare occurrence, as the body requires this amino acid for proper functioning. However, in certain cases such as genetic disorders or severely restricted diets, deficiency symptoms may include fatigue, irritability, and decreased immunity. Conversely, excessive doses of tryptophan may lead to toxicity symptoms, including nausea, vomiting, and diarrhea.

Caution is advised when using tryptophan in conjunction with certain medications, such as antidepressants, as interactions may occur. Additionally, individuals with a history of liver or kidney disease should use tryptophan cautiously, given these organs' role in amino acid metabolism.

Candidates suitable for tryptophan infusion include those who are malnourished or facing challenges in nutrient absorption, as well as individuals with mood or sleep-related conditions such as depression or insomnia. Tryptophan may be combined with other compounds and amino acids in IV hydration solutions to enhance its therapeutic effects.

The frequency of tryptophan infusion varies based on patient-specific needs and therapy goals, typically ranging from 1-2 grams per day for adults. Infusions may be administered daily or several times per week, aligning with individual requirements.

Clinical information about tryptophan includes its various forms—found in protein-rich foods and available as supplements in capsules, tablets, and powders. Storage recommendations emphasize a cool, dry place away from direct sunlight and heat, and preparation for IV infusion involves reconstitution with sterile water or saline solution.

Tryptophan's therapeutic potential has been explored in conditions such as depression, anxiety, and sleep disorders. However, optimal dosage and duration of supplementation vary and depend on individual response to treatment. For instance, treatment protocols for depression may involve daily doses of 1-2 grams of tryptophan for up to 12 weeks, while sleep disorder protocols may recommend a single dose of 1-2 grams before bedtime.

The half-life of tryptophan is relatively short, approximately 2-3 hours, suggesting a rapid decline in levels under conditions of high oxidative stress or toxin exposure. Despite being a stable compound unaffected by heat, light, or air, proper storage is recommended to maintain maximal potency and efficacy.

Valine

Valine, classified as an essential amino acid, assumes a pivotal role in critical physiological processes such as protein synthesis, muscle growth and repair, and energy production. As one of the three branched-chain amino acids (BCAAs), alongside leucine and isoleucine, valine contributes significantly to the intricate network of bodily functions. Although not typically utilized as the primary component in IV hydration solutions, valine can be introduced into these solutions to offer supplementary nutritional support in specific contexts.

The multifaceted benefits of valine encompass its integral role in muscle growth and repair, regulation of blood sugar levels, provision of energy, potential positive impact on immune function, and contribution to wound healing processes. Dosage recommendations for valine in IV infusion hinge on individual patient needs and therapeutic objectives, with typical dosages ranging from 2 to 4 grams per day for adults. It is crucial to note that excessive valine doses may lead to toxicity.

While valine is not frequently employed as a standalone therapy for specific medical conditions, its inclusion in IV hydration solutions is considered in situations requiring additional nutritional support. This may include cases of malnourishment or conditions affecting nutrient absorption from food. Valine deficiency is rare, given its essential role in proper bodily function, yet it may manifest in certain circumstances such as genetic disorders or severely restricted diets, presenting symptoms like fatigue, weakness, and compromised immune function.

Valine toxicity, resulting from excessive doses, may induce symptoms such as nausea, vomiting, and diarrhea. Caution is advised when considering valine infusion for patients with a history of liver or kidney disease, as these organs play a crucial role in amino acid metabolism.

Potential candidates for valine infusion encompass malnourished individuals, those with conditions affecting nutrient absorption, and athletes or individuals engaged in intense physical activity as part of a broader IV hydration solution.

Valine may be employed in conjunction with other compounds and amino acids in IV hydration solutions, potentially combined with other BCAAs to enhance nutritional support. The frequency of valine infusion is tailored to individual patient needs, with typical dosages ranging from 2 to 4 grams per day for adults, administered daily or several times per week.

Clinical information on valine covers its various forms, daily dosage limits, storage instructions, preparation for IV infusion, treatment protocols, and half-life considerations. Valine, found in protein-rich foods and available in supplement forms such as capsules, tablets, and powders, lacks an established daily dosage limit due to its essential nature for normal growth and development.

Valine supplements should be stored in a cool, dry place, shielded from direct sunlight and heat, to maintain maximal potency and efficacy. The half-life of valine in the body is relatively short, approximately 3-4 hours, highlighting the potential for rapid declines in valine levels under conditions of high oxidative stress or toxin exposure. Valine is a stable compound, resilient to the effects of heat, light, or air, but adherence to proper storage guidelines ensures its optimal effectiveness.

Nonessential Amino Acids in IV Hydration

Alanine

Alanine, classified as a non-essential amino acid, assumes a pivotal role in fundamental physiological processes such as energy production, immune function, and glucose metabolism. Abundantly present in the body, alanine is synthesized from pyruvate in the liver. Although not typically the primary constituent of IV hydration solutions, it can be judiciously incorporated to offer supplementary nutritional support under specific circumstances.

The multifaceted benefits of alanine encompass its role as a precursor to glucose production, contributing significantly to the body's energy production. Furthermore, alanine plays a crucial part in bolstering the immune system, facilitating antibody production, and regulating immune responses. Additionally, it may contribute to diminishing muscle breakdown during exercise, thereby potentially enhancing overall exercise performance.

The appropriate dosage of alanine for IV infusion is contingent upon the patient's specific needs and therapy goals, typically ranging from 2-4 grams per day for adults. It is imperative to note that excessive doses of alanine can be toxic.

While alanine is not commonly employed as a standalone therapy for specific medical conditions, its inclusion in IV hydration solutions can be considered for patients facing malnutrition or conditions impeding nutrient absorption. The rarity of alanine deficiency stems from the body's capacity to synthesize it from other amino acids. However, in instances such as liver disease or severe dietary restrictions, deficiency symptoms may manifest as fatigue, weakness, and compromised immune function.

Conversely, excessive doses of alanine may result in toxicity, leading to symptoms such as nausea, vomiting, and diarrhea. Caution should be exercised in patients with a history of liver or kidney disease, as these organs are crucial for amino acid metabolism.

Patients susceptible to malnutrition or with conditions affecting nutrient absorption, as well as athletes or individuals engaged in intense physical activity, are identified as potential candidates for alanine infusion. The possibility of combining alanine with other compounds and amino acids in IV hydration solutions, such as glutamine and arginine, is explored to provide comprehensive nutritional support.

The frequency of alanine infusion depends on individual patient needs and therapy goals, with typical dosages administered daily or several times per week.

Clinical information elucidates that alanine is naturally found in protein-rich foods like meat, fish, and dairy products, with supplements available in various forms. Storage recommendations emphasize a cool, dry place away from direct sunlight and heat. Preparation for IV infusion involves reconstituting alanine with sterile water or saline solution, ensuring immediate use or refrigeration for later use to maintain efficacy.

The book further delves into treatment protocols, exploring potential therapeutic benefits in muscle growth and repair, glucose metabolism, and immune function. Despite ongoing research, establishing optimal dosage and duration for alanine supplementation remains a dynamic field, dependent on individual response and health conditions.

The half-life of alanine is relatively short, approximately 1-3 hours, making its levels susceptible to rapid decline under conditions of high oxidative stress or toxin exposure. Stability analysis reveals that while alanine is generally resistant to heat, light, and air, prudent storage measures are necessary to preserve its efficacy.

In conclusion, the intricate exploration of alanine in the book encompasses its physiological significance, dosage considerations, potential applications in IV hydration therapy, clinical implications, and storage protocols. This comprehensive guide caters to healthcare professionals, patients seeking alternative treatments, and individuals interested in understanding the nuanced role of alanine in health and wellness.

Arginine

Arginine, classified as a semi-essential amino acid, assumes a pivotal role in numerous physiological processes, contributing to wound healing, immune function, and cardiovascular health. As a precursor to nitric oxide, it regulates blood flow and plays a vital role in the immune response. While not typically employed as the primary component of IV hydration solutions, arginine can be strategically added to such solutions to provide supplementary nutritional support in specific circumstances.

The multifaceted benefits of arginine encompass its critical role in wound healing, immune function, and its contribution as a precursor to nitric oxide. Additionally, arginine exhibits potential in improving cardiovascular health, enhancing exercise performance, and fostering the growth of lean body mass. Dosage recommendations for arginine in IV infusion are contingent upon individual patient needs and therapeutic goals, typically ranging from 6-30 grams per day for adults. It is essential to exercise caution as excessive doses may lead to toxicity.

Arginine may be integrated into IV hydration solutions to offer additional nutritional support for patients experiencing malnutrition, conditions affecting nutrient absorption, or those in recovery from surgery or injury. While arginine deficiency is rare due to the body's ability to synthesize it from other amino acids, specific instances, such as in patients with liver disease or on severely restricted diets, may result in deficiency symptoms like fatigue, weakness, and decreased immune function. Conversely, excessive doses of arginine may induce toxicity, manifesting as nausea, vomiting, and diarrhea.

Patients with a history of liver or kidney disease should exercise caution when using arginine, as these organs are responsible for amino acid metabolism. Moreover, potential interactions with medications such as blood pressure medications, diabetes medications, and nitrates necessitate careful consideration. Candidates for arginine infusion include malnourished individuals, post-surgery or injury recovery patients, and those with conditions impacting nutrient absorption. Athletes or individuals undergoing intense physical activity may also derive benefits from arginine infusion within a comprehensive IV hydration solution.

Arginine's potential synergy with other compounds and amino acids in IV hydration solutions is explored, highlighting its possible combination with amino acids like glutamine and citrulline for enhanced nutritional support. The frequency of arginine infusion is tailored to the patient's needs, typically administered daily or several times per week.

The clinical information section provides insights into the various forms of arginine, daily dosage limits, storage recommendations, and preparation for IV infusion. Treatment protocols for specific health conditions, such as cardiovascular disease and erectile dysfunction, are discussed, emphasizing the need for individualized approaches. Arginine's relatively short half-life, stability, and storage considerations are also addressed, ensuring maximal potency and efficacy.

In conclusion, this comprehensive guide offers a nuanced exploration of arginine's role in IV hydration therapy, catering to healthcare professionals, patients seeking alternative treatments, and those intrigued by innovative health strategies. With a focus on evidence-based information, the book equips readers with the knowledge to make informed decisions, maximizing the potential benefits of arginine within the realm of IV hydration therapy.

Glutamine

Glutamine, classified as a non-essential amino acid, assumes paramount importance in fortifying the immune system and maintaining intestinal health. Integral to energy production and the preservation of intestinal lining integrity, glutamine often constitutes a pivotal component in IV hydration solutions, providing enhanced nutritional support in specific scenarios.

The multifaceted benefits of glutamine encompass its role in immune system fortification, intestinal health maintenance, energy production facilitation, and potential improvement in muscle mass and exercise performance. Dosage recommendations for glutamine in IV infusion hinge on patient-specific needs and therapeutic goals, typically ranging from 5-20 grams per day for adults. However, careful consideration is paramount to avoid toxic doses.

Glutamine's therapeutic applications extend to IV hydration solutions for patients contending with malnutrition, conditions hindering nutrient absorption, or those convalescing from surgery or injury. Furthermore, glutamine may find utility in treating certain gastrointestinal disorders, such as inflammatory bowel disease.

While glutamine deficiency is rare due to the body's ability to synthesize it from other amino acids, instances may arise in severe burns or trauma, manifesting as fatigue, weakness, and compromised immune function. Conversely, excessive glutamine doses may induce toxicity, resulting in symptoms like nausea, vomiting, and diarrhea.

Caution is advised in patients with a history of liver or kidney disease, as these organs metabolize amino acids. Additionally, interactions with certain medications, including anti-epileptic drugs and antibiotics, warrant consideration.

Prime candidates for glutamine infusion include malnourished individuals, postoperative or injury-recovering patients, and those with conditions impacting nutrient absorption. Athletes engaged in intense physical activity may also benefit from glutamine infusion within a broader IV hydration solution.

The potential coadministration of glutamine with other compounds and amino acids in IV therapy, such as arginine and citrulline, is explored, providing additional nutritional support.

Frequency of glutamine infusion aligns with patient-specific needs, typically ranging from 5-20 grams per day for adults, with administration frequencies determined by therapeutic goals.

Clinical information underscores the varied forms of glutamine, including powder, capsule, and liquid, its daily dosage limits contingent on factors like age and health status, appropriate storage practices, and preparation for IV infusion with sterile water or saline solution. Treatment protocols highlight glutamine's studied therapeutic benefits across critical illness, cancer, and inflammatory bowel disease, emphasizing the need for individualized approaches.

The half-life of glutamine is relatively short, approximately 15 minutes, necessitating continuous replenishment through dietary sources or supplementation. Despite its stability in the face of heat and light, glutamine exhibits sensitivity to moisture, emphasizing the importance of proper storage practices to ensure maximal potency and efficacy.

Glycine

Glycine, a non-essential amino acid, plays a pivotal role in various physiological processes as a fundamental building block of proteins and a key participant in metabolic pathways within the body. The book extensively explores the multifaceted benefits of glycine, ranging from its contribution to improved sleep quality and reduced sleep onset latency to its potential support for cognitive function, memory enhancement in older adults, and promotion of healthy skin and joints.

Dosage recommendations for glycine in the context of IV hydration therapy are nuanced, dependent on factors such as age, weight, and medical history. Clinical studies have observed doses ranging from 10 to 30 grams per day, reflecting the variability in individual requirements.

Glycine has been the subject of research as a potential treatment for various medical conditions, including sleep disorders, cognitive decline, and joint pain. Deficiency in glycine, although rare given its non-essential nature, may manifest in symptoms such as fatigue, muscle weakness, poor sleep quality, and cognitive impairment. The book delves into signs of both deficiency and toxicity, emphasizing the generally safe nature of glycine when used as directed, with potential side effects primarily associated with high doses.

Contraindications are minimal, and glycine infusion is generally considered safe. However, individuals with specific medical conditions, such as kidney disease, are advised to consult with healthcare professionals before incorporating glycine into their regimen.

The book identifies potential candidates who may benefit from glycine infusion, including those with sleep disorders, cognitive decline, or joint pain. Glycine may be used in combination with other amino acids and compounds in IV hydration therapy, enhancing its therapeutic effects, as illustrated by the tri-amino blend comprising glycine, arginine, and methionine.

Treatment frequency varies, with some cases warranting daily infusions for a specified period, while others may require less frequent administration. Duration of treatment is tailored to the patient's condition and response to therapy.

Clinical information on glycine encompasses its various forms, daily dosage limits, storage considerations, and preparation for IV infusion. Additionally, treatment protocols shed light on the diverse therapeutic benefits glycine may offer in conditions such as schizophrenia, sleep disorders, and muscle damage. The book underscores the importance of glycine's relatively short half-life of approximately four hours, necessitating continuous replenishment through dietary sources or supplementation.

In summary, glycine emerges as a stable and soluble compound with potential therapeutic benefits, its comprehensive exploration providing valuable insights for healthcare professionals, patients seeking alternative treatments, and those interested in the nuanced aspects of IV hydration therapy. The book serves as a crucial resource for individuals looking to enhance their understanding of glycine and its role in promoting optimal health and well-being.

Amino Acid Derivatives Used In IV Hydration

Glutathione

Glutathione, a tripeptide composed of three amino acids—glutamine, cysteine, and glycine—is a pivotal antioxidant and detoxifier within the human body. Its role in safeguarding cells from damage induced by free radicals and other harmful substances is fundamental. The book thoroughly explores the multifaceted benefits of glutathione, ranging from its potent antioxidant activity to its crucial involvement in the body's detoxification processes, immune support, and potential contributions to skin health.

The recommended dosage of glutathione for IV hydration therapy is contingent upon factors such as the patient's age, weight, and medical history. Clinical studies have utilized doses ranging from 250 to 1,500 milligrams per day. Glutathione has shown potential benefits for individuals with various health conditions, including chronic fatigue syndrome, Parkinson's disease, Alzheimer's disease, multiple sclerosis, rheumatoid arthritis, inflammatory bowel disease, chronic obstructive pulmonary disease (COPD), asthma, cardiovascular disease, liver disease, diabetes, and cancer. Moreover, it may prove advantageous for athletes or bodybuilders, aiding in reducing muscle damage, fatigue, and supporting post-workout recovery.

The book delves into the detailed exploration of glutathione's potential efficacy in treating specific medical conditions, such as Parkinson's disease, liver disease, and respiratory diseases like asthma and COPD. Despite glutathione deficiency being rare due to the body's ability to produce it, signs may include increased oxidative stress, impaired immune function, and an elevated risk of chronic diseases.

While generally considered safe when used as directed, high doses of glutathione may result in side effects such as nausea, vomiting, and diarrhea. Special considerations are outlined for individuals with asthma or allergies, those undergoing chemotherapy, and those with pre-existing kidney disease.

Determining good candidates for glutathione infusion involves a case-by-case evaluation by healthcare professionals, with potential benefits for individuals with Parkinson's disease, liver disease, or respiratory diseases. The coadministration of glutathione with other compounds or amino acids in IV therapy is explored, emphasizing individualized treatment protocols.

The book provides insights into the frequency of glutathione infusion treatments, with standard doses ranging from 300mg to 1,500mg per session, depending on the individual's health condition and treatment goals. Special notes highlight the light sensitivity of glutathione, necessitating careful storage and administration to maintain its potency.

Clinical information encompasses various aspects, including the forms of glutathione, daily dosage limits, storage guidelines, preparation for IV infusion, treatment protocols, the half-life of glutathione, and its stability. Overall, this comprehensive guide serves as an invaluable resource for healthcare professionals, patients, and those interested in the intricate details of utilizing glutathione in IV hydration therapy for optimal health and wellness.

Taurine

Taurine, classified as a non-essential amino acid, assumes a pivotal role in numerous physiological processes within the body. Its significance extends to supporting cardiovascular health, regulating electrolyte balance, modulating the immune system, and fostering antioxidant activity. Within the context of IV hydration therapy, taurine supplementation holds promise for enhancing exercise performance, cognitive function, and alleviating symptoms associated with certain health conditions.

The recommended dosage of taurine for IV hydration is contingent upon individual health needs and treatment objectives. Generally falling within the range of 500mg to 2,000mg per session, these doses are tailored to specific health goals. Taurine finds application as an adjunct therapy for diverse health conditions, encompassing cardiovascular disease, diabetes, liver disease, neurological disorders, and as a support for athletic performance and recovery.

While taurine deficiency is rare in those maintaining a balanced diet, certain health conditions may elevate the risk, leading to symptoms such as impaired vision, muscle weakness, fatigue, and cognitive dysfunction. On the contrary, excessive taurine intake, though generally considered safe when used as directed, may result in gastrointestinal upset and, in rare instances, neurological symptoms such as seizures or confusion.

Contraindications merit attention, especially concerning potential interactions with medications like lithium and blood pressure medications. Caution is advised in individuals with a history of kidney or liver disease, and its use during pregnancy and breastfeeding is discouraged due to limited research on safety in these populations. For those with kidney disease, the excretion of taurine by the kidneys raises concerns of potential accumulation and subsequent toxicity.

Taurine infusion is considered beneficial for individuals with specific health conditions such as cardiovascular or liver disease, and it may prove advantageous for athletes or those seeking to enhance exercise performance and cognitive function. The potential synergistic effects of taurine in combination with other amino acids or compounds, such as glutathione or vitamin B12, are explored, highlighting its versatility in supporting overall health and wellness.

The frequency of taurine IV hydration treatments is flexible, varying based on individual health needs and response to treatment. Some may undergo weekly or bi-weekly sessions, while others may require treatments at different intervals.

Clinical information supplements the discussion, addressing the various forms of taurine, daily dosage limits, storage requirements, preparation for IV infusion, and treatment protocols. While taurine is generally stable and well-tolerated, its short half-life necessitates careful consideration under conditions of high oxidative stress or toxin exposure.

This comprehensive exploration of taurine within the realm of IV hydration therapy provides valuable insights for healthcare professionals, patients, and individuals seeking to optimize their health and well-being.

Carnitine

Carnitine, an amino acid integral to energy production and metabolism, assumes a pivotal role in the transport of fatty acids into mitochondria—crucial for their conversion into ATP, the body's primary energy source. The book explores the manifold benefits of carnitine supplementation via intravenous (IV) hydration, potentially encompassing improved athletic performance, enhanced weight loss, and alleviation of symptoms associated with certain health conditions.

Dosing recommendations for IV carnitine therapy hinge on individual health needs and treatment objectives, typically ranging from 500mg to 2,000mg per session. Carnitine's applicability as an adjunct therapy extends to diverse health conditions such as heart disease, peripheral artery disease, and type 2 diabetes. It may also support athletic performance and weight loss endeavors.

While carnitine deficiency is rare in individuals with a balanced diet, certain health conditions, such as liver or kidney disease, may elevate the risk. Deficiency symptoms include muscle weakness, fatigue, and impaired exercise performance. Carnitine toxicity is generally considered safe when used as directed, but high doses may lead to gastrointestinal upset, seizures, or hypoglycemia in rare instances.

Contraindications involve potential interactions with specific medications and caution for individuals with a history of seizures or kidney disease due to the possibility of exacerbation. The book identifies individuals with health conditions such as heart disease or type 2 diabetes, as well as athletes or those seeking improved exercise performance or weight loss, as potential candidates for carnitine infusion.

Carnitine's synergy with other compounds or amino acids, such as taurine or glutamine, is explored, highlighting its role in comprehensive IV hydration therapies. The frequency of IV carnitine treatments varies based on individual health needs and responses to treatment, with some individuals receiving weekly or bi-weekly sessions.

Clinical information provides a deeper understanding of carnitine, covering its various forms, daily dosage considerations, storage guidelines, preparation for IV infusion, treatment protocols, half-life, and stability. The book delves into the potential therapeutic benefits of carnitine for heart disease, diabetes, and neurological disorders, while emphasizing the necessity of professional guidance due to varying optimal dosages for different health conditions. The relatively short half-life of carnitine, approximately 4-6 hours, underlines the importance of timely administration.

Carnitine, deemed a stable compound unaffected by heat, light, or air, is recommended for storage in cool, dry places away from direct sunlight and heat to ensure maximal potency and efficacy. This comprehensive guide serves as an invaluable resource for healthcare professionals, patients exploring alternative treatments, or individuals intrigued by the potential of IV hydration therapies featuring carnitine. The transformative potential of such therapies, when coupled with the knowledge provided in this book, becomes a promising avenue for optimizing health and well-being.

Orthinine

Ornithine, a non-essential amino acid derivative, assumes a pivotal role in the urea cycle and the synthesis of nitric oxide within the body. This comprehensive exploration delves into the multifaceted aspects of ornithine, particularly its application in Intravenous (IV) hydration therapy and its potential benefits. Ornithine is recognized for its potential to support muscle growth, enhance athletic performance, alleviate fatigue, and expedite wound healing when administered through IV therapy.

The recommended dosage of ornithine for IV hydration is contingent upon individual health needs and treatment objectives, with typical doses ranging from 1,000mg to 5,000mg per session. Ornithine emerges as an adjunct therapy for an array of health conditions, including liver disease, urea cycle disorders, and hormone imbalances. Moreover, it has garnered attention for its utility in supporting athletic performance, reducing fatigue, and facilitating wound healing.

While ornithine deficiency is rare in individuals adhering to a balanced diet, specific health conditions, such as liver disease or urea cycle disorders, may elevate the risk of deficiency. Indicators of ornithine deficiency encompass fatigue, muscle weakness, and impaired athletic performance. Conversely, ornithine toxicity is generally considered rare when used as directed, although high doses may result in gastrointestinal upset, including nausea, vomiting, and diarrhea, with rare instances of hypotension or seizures.

This detailed examination underscores contraindications, where ornithine may interact with certain medications, including antipsychotics and benzodiazepines. Caution is warranted for individuals with a history of seizures or liver disease due to the potential exacerbation of these conditions with high ornithine doses.

Identifying suitable candidates for ornithine infusion encompasses individuals with specific health conditions like liver disease or urea cycle disorders, as well as athletes or those aiming to improve exercise performance, reduce fatigue, or enhance wound healing. Ornithine may be used synergistically with other amino acids or compounds, such as arginine or citrulline, in IV therapy to augment its therapeutic effects and support overall health and wellness.

The frequency of ornithine IV hydration treatments is contingent upon individual health needs and responsiveness to treatment, with variations in treatment frequency from weekly to bi-weekly or less frequent administration.

Clinical information delves into the diverse forms ornithine supplements are available in, daily dosage considerations, proper storage practices, preparation for IV infusion, and pertinent treatment protocols for various health conditions. Ornithine, although synthesized by the body, offers potential therapeutic benefits that are still under investigation, with optimal dosage and duration contingent upon individual responses and health conditions.

The half-life of ornithine in the body is notably short, approximately 25 minutes, signifying its rapid decline under conditions of heightened oxidative stress or toxin exposure. Ornithine is considered a stable compound, unaffected by heat, light, or air; however, adherence to proper storage practices ensures maximal potency and efficacy.

This comprehensive elucidation on ornithine within the context of IV hydration therapy serves as an invaluable resource for healthcare professionals, patients seeking alternative treatments, and individuals interested in exploring innovative approaches to health and well-being.

Citrulline

Citrulline, a non-essential amino acid derivative, assumes a pivotal role in the urea cycle and the synthesis of nitric oxide. This intricate molecule finds application in Intravenous (IV) hydration therapy, where it can potentially support athletic performance, mitigate fatigue, and bolster immune function.

The recommended dosage of citrulline for IV hydration is contingent upon individual health needs and treatment objectives, typically ranging from 1,000mg to 5,000mg per session. Citrulline may serve as an adjunct therapy for various health conditions, including cardiovascular disease, erectile dysfunction, and muscle wasting. Additionally, it proves beneficial for athletes or those aiming to enhance exercise performance, alleviate fatigue, or fortify immune function.

While citrulline deficiency is rare in individuals with a balanced diet, specific health conditions such as urea cycle disorders or liver disease may elevate the risk. Deficiency signs include fatigue, muscle weakness, and compromised immune function. Citrulline is generally safe, but high doses may induce gastrointestinal upset, and in rare instances, hypotension or seizures.

Caution is advised regarding potential interactions with medications like nitrates and phosphodiesterase inhibitors. Individuals with a history of hypotension or liver disease should also exercise caution, as high doses might exacerbate these conditions.

Ideal candidates for citrulline infusion include those with cardiovascular disease, erectile dysfunction, muscle wasting, athletes, or individuals seeking improved exercise performance, reduced fatigue, or enhanced immune function. Citrulline may be combined with other amino acids or compounds, such as arginine or ornithine, to amplify its therapeutic effects. Furthermore, it may be integrated into comprehensive IV hydration therapies to support overall health and wellness.

The frequency of citrulline IV hydration treatments is tailored to individual health needs and treatment responses. Some individuals may receive weekly or bi-weekly treatments, while others may undergo treatments more or less frequently.

Clinical information pertaining to citrulline encompasses its various forms (capsules, tablets, powders, and liquid), absence of a daily dosage limit, proper storage conditions (cool, dry place, away from sunlight and heat), preparation for IV infusion (reconstitution with sterile water or saline solution), and treatment protocols. Studies have explored citrulline's potential therapeutic benefits in heart disease, hypertension, and erectile dysfunction, with varied dosages and durations.

Citrulline exhibits a relatively short half-life of approximately 1-2 hours, making its levels susceptible to rapid decline under conditions of high oxidative stress or toxin exposure. Despite being a stable compound unaffected by heat, light, or air, proper storage in suitable conditions is essential for ensuring maximal potency and efficacy.

In conclusion, this comprehensive exploration of citrulline in IV hydration therapy provides valuable insights for healthcare professionals, patients, and individuals interested in optimizing their health and well-being.

N-acetylcysteine (NAC)

N-acetylcysteine (NAC), a derivative of the naturally occurring amino acid cysteine, holds significant importance as a potent antioxidant and a precursor to glutathione—an essential antioxidant within the body. This compound has been extensively utilized both as a supplement and a pharmaceutical drug, demonstrating a wide range of potential health-related benefits.

The multifaceted advantages of NAC encompass antioxidant support, wherein it aids in replenishing glutathione levels, thereby safeguarding cells from oxidative stress. Additionally, NAC plays a pivotal role in promoting respiratory health by thinning mucus and reducing inflammation, offering protection to the liver by facilitating detoxification and preventing damage from toxic substances. Moreover, it exhibits promise in contributing to mental health improvements, potentially alleviating symptoms of depression, anxiety, and other psychiatric disorders. Furthermore, NAC holds potential in providing neurological support and safeguarding against neurodegenerative diseases such as Alzheimer's and Parkinson's.

The dosage of NAC in IV therapy is contingent upon the specific condition being treated and the individual patient's needs, typically ranging from 600 to 1800 mg per infusion. Higher doses may be administered under medical supervision. NAC has been applied in the treatment of various conditions, including chronic obstructive pulmonary disease (COPD), asthma, acetaminophen (paracetamol) poisoning, liver diseases, mental health disorders, chronic fatigue syndrome, and immune system support.

While there is no established deficiency state for NAC itself, low levels of glutathione, the antioxidant replenished by NAC, can lead to increased oxidative stress, potentially contributing to various health issues. Generally considered safe, NAC may cause side effects such as nausea, vomiting, diarrhea, abdominal pain, and headaches with excessive intake. Contraindications for NAC include certain medical conditions or medications, making it unsuitable for individuals with asthma, kidney or liver disease, bleeding disorders, or active infections.

Ideal candidates for NAC infusion are individuals with conditions known to benefit from NAC treatment, such as respiratory issues, liver diseases, or psychiatric disorders, and who have no contraindications. NAC can be administered alone or in combination with other vitamins, minerals, and antioxidants in IV therapy, tailored to specific treatment goals and patient needs.

The frequency of NAC treatments varies based on the condition being treated and individual response to therapy, typically administered once or twice a week initially, with adjustments made as necessary. Various clinical aspects of NAC are explored, including its forms, daily dosage limits, storage conditions, preparation for IV infusion, treatment protocols, half-life considerations, and stability.

NAC's availability in various forms, including oral capsules, tablets, effervescent tablets, and intravenous (IV) solutions, contributes to its versatility. The recommended daily dosage for oral use ranges from 600 to 1,800 mg per day, divided into two or three doses, while IV dosage is determined by a healthcare professional based on the specific condition being treated.

Proper storage of NAC at room temperature in a dry, cool place away from direct sunlight ensures its stability. NAC is typically prepared for IV infusion by mixing the appropriate dose in a sterile saline solution or another compatible IV fluid. The therapeutic benefits of NAC in various health conditions have been studied, yet the optimal dosage and duration of supplementation may vary depending on individual needs and response to treatment.

In conclusion, this detailed exploration of N-acetylcysteine underscores its diverse benefits, potential applications, and the nuanced considerations that underpin its use in IV therapy, providing a comprehensive resource for healthcare professionals and those seeking a deeper understanding of this valuable compound.

Summary

The significance of amino acids in various physiological processes, encompassing muscle growth and repair, immune function, and energy production, cannot be overstated. While the body synthesizes some amino acids, others are acquired through dietary sources or supplements. The roster of crucial amino acids, such as L-Leucine, L-Lysine, L-Methionine, L-Glutamine, L-Arginine, L-Carnitine, L-Cysteine, L-Ornithine, L-Taurine, and L-Citrulline, underscores their diverse roles within the body.

Amino acid supplementation holds potential benefits for individuals with specific medical conditions, as well as for athletes and those seeking to optimize exercise performance and recovery. However, caution is imperative, especially in patients with liver conditions, as the liver is the primary site of amino acid metabolism. Excessive levels can lead to toxicity, characterized by symptoms such as nausea, vomiting, and diarrhea.

Amino acid lab testing, a valuable tool for monitoring levels, should be conducted judiciously and in collaboration with healthcare professionals. Interpretation of these test results demands specialized expertise in biochemistry, nutrition, and clinical medicine. Professionals with specialized training, including clinical biochemists, nutritionists, and medical geneticists, are best equipped to navigate the intricacies of amino acid level testing.

The complexity of interpreting amino acid levels necessitates a comprehensive evaluation, considering the patient's overall health, clinical history, dietary habits, and potential metabolic disorders. Elevated levels of specific amino acids may signal an underlying metabolic disorder, while low levels may indicate nutritional deficiencies or other health issues. Furthermore, the interpretation must be contextualized within the patient's broader healthcare landscape, involving the integration of other laboratory tests and diagnostic imaging studies for a holistic understanding. In essence, the nuanced interpretation of amino acid levels is an integral component of personalized healthcare, requiring a multidisciplinary approach for accurate and meaningful insights.

CHAPTER SEVEN
COENZYMES

Enzymes, indispensable proteins in living organisms, play a pivotal role in accelerating biochemical reactions essential for various physiological processes, including digestion, metabolism, and energy production. However, the intricate orchestration of these enzymatic activities necessitates the collaborative involvement of coenzymes, small organic non-protein molecules that act as crucial partners to enzymes.

Coenzymes, acting as facilitators, are instrumental in enzymatic activities by serving as carriers for chemical groups or electrons during the intricate choreography of biochemical reactions. A compelling example is the coenzyme nicotinamide adenine dinucleotide (NAD+), which adeptly shuttles electrons between molecules in the cellular respiration process, ultimately generating energy for cellular functions. It is noteworthy that numerous coenzymes, vital for these intricate processes, trace their origins back to essential vitamins, exemplified by the vitamin B complex and vitamin C. A case in point is pyridoxal phosphate (PLP), a coenzyme derived from vitamin B6, actively involved in amino acid metabolism. Another illustrative coenzyme is coenzyme Q10, derived from vitamin K, playing a crucial role in the electron transport chain within mitochondria, where cellular energy is generated.

Coenzymes, characterized by their transient binding with enzymes during catalytic processes, distinguish themselves by their ability to be utilized by multiple enzymes. This inherent versatility enhances the efficiency of resource utilization. Moreover, the temporary nature of their binding allows coenzymes to be readily regenerated after the completion of a reaction, often through subsequent series of reactions, rendering them available for reuse in subsequent biochemical activities.

Essentially, coenzymes emerge as indispensable molecules working in tandem with enzymes to catalyze and regulate complex biochemical reactions within living organisms. With their capacity to temporarily bind to enzymes, carry vital chemical groups or electrons, and derive from essential vitamins, coenzymes represent a dynamic and essential component of cellular processes. Their ability to be regenerated for subsequent reuse further underscores their efficiency and significance in the intricate dance of biochemical reactions.

Coenzyme Q10

Coenzyme Q10 (CoQ10), also recognized as ubiquinone, is an inherent, fat-soluble compound pervasive in nearly every cell of the human body. Its paramount role in the mitochondrial electron transport chain underscores its significance in generating adenosine triphosphate (ATP), the primary cellular energy source. CoQ10 assumes the additional role of an antioxidant, safeguarding cells from oxidative stress and free radical damage. The book illuminates the intricate relationship between CoQ10 levels and vitamin deficiencies, particularly emphasizing the contributions of vitamin B2 (riboflavin), vitamin B6 (pyridoxine), and vitamin C to CoQ10 synthesis.

A deficit in riboflavin, for instance, can diminish CoQ10 production, as riboflavin is integral to its synthesis. Similarly, a deficiency in vitamin B6 can impact CoQ10 levels, given its involvement in the conversion of CoQ10 from its precursor, ubiquinone. Conversely, certain studies suggest that supplementation with vitamins E and C may elevate CoQ10 levels by preventing its degradation and facilitating its regeneration.

The book outlines an array of benefits attributed to CoQ10, including support for cellular energy production, promotion of heart health, potential mitigation of muscle pain associated with statin use, enhancement of fertility, cognitive function support, and potential symptom improvement in conditions such as Parkinson's and Huntington's diseases.

Dosage recommendations are contingent on factors such as age, health status, and the specific condition being treated, typically ranging from 30 to 200 mg per day, with higher dosages up to 1200 mg per day under medical supervision. Conditions addressed with CoQ10 encompass congestive heart failure, high blood pressure, migraines, mitochondrial disorders, age-related macular degeneration, and Parkinson's disease.

Signs of CoQ10 deficiency manifest as fatigue, muscle weakness and pain, cognitive difficulties, and weakened immune system. CoQ10 toxicity is rare but may result in mild symptoms such as nausea, diarrhea, heartburn, or insomnia. Contraindications include caution for individuals on blood-thinning medications like warfarin and pregnant or nursing women.

The book identifies good candidates for CoQ10 infusion, including those with congestive heart failure, mitochondrial disorders, individuals undergoing statin therapy, and those experiencing fatigue or age-related cognitive decline. It also explores CoQ10's combination with other nutrients and compounds in IV therapy, such as B vitamins, vitamin C, and glutathione, to enhance overall health and wellness.

Detailed clinical information covers various aspects of CoQ10, including its forms, daily dosage limits, storage instructions, preparation for IV infusion, treatment protocols, half-life considerations, and stability. This comprehensive guide serves as an invaluable resource for healthcare professionals, patients seeking alternative treatments, and those intrigued by innovative health approaches. The transformative potential of CoQ10, when understood through the knowledge imparted in this book, offers a pathway to enhanced health and well-being across a spectrum of conditions.

Nicotinamide Adenine Dinucleotide (NAD+)

Nicotinamide Adenine Dinucleotide (NAD+) stands as a pivotal coenzyme in a multitude of biochemical reactions within the human body. Its primary role lies in energy metabolism, where it actively participates in the production of adenosine triphosphate (ATP), the principal energy source for cellular functions. Functioning as an electron and hydrogen ion carrier, NAD+ is instrumental in various metabolic processes, including glycolysis, the Krebs cycle, and oxidative phosphorylation.

In glycolysis, NAD+ undergoes reduction to NADH, transporting electrons generated during glucose breakdown. In the Krebs cycle, NAD+ contributes to the conversion of pyruvate to ATP. In oxidative phosphorylation, NADH is oxidized back to NAD+, yielding ATP. Beyond its role in energy metabolism, NAD+ plays a crucial part in DNA repair, gene expression, and cell signaling, acting as a key regulator of cellular homeostasis.

However, NAD+ levels are subject to influences such as diet, exercise, stress, and age. Research indicates a decline in NAD+ levels with age, potentially contributing to age-related diseases and diminished cellular function. Supplementation with NAD+ precursors, such as nicotinamide riboside (NR), has demonstrated the ability to elevate NAD+ levels, offering various health benefits. NR, a form of vitamin B3, converts to NAD+ in the body, leading to improved energy metabolism, enhanced mitochondrial function, and reduced inflammation.

As a coenzyme integral to cellular processes, NAD+ assumes a crucial role in maintaining the integrity of our DNA, ensuring proper functionality, and regulating biological processes. Unfortunately, aging results in a decreased production of NAD+, posing potential issues.

The benefits of NAD+ encompass improved energy metabolism, heightened mitochondrial function, reduced inflammation, and enhanced cognitive function. NAD+ has demonstrated neuroprotective effects, improved athletic performance, and support for detoxification pathways. Dosage recommendations for IV administration of NAD+ vary based on individual needs and health conditions, typically ranging from 250 to 1000 mg per infusion, administered under healthcare professional supervision.

NAD+ infusion therapy finds application in treating conditions such as addiction, chronic fatigue syndrome, fibromyalgia, neurodegenerative disorders, and mitochondrial disorders. It has also been used as a complementary therapy for cancer patients undergoing chemotherapy.

Signs of NAD+ deficiency include fatigue, decreased physical and mental performance, and an increased risk of chronic diseases. While signs of NAD+ toxicity are rare, they may include flushing, dizziness, nausea, and headache. Contraindications for NAD+ infusion therapy include severe liver or kidney disease, certain genetic disorders, and it is contraindicated for pregnant or breastfeeding women.

Ideal candidates for NAD+ infusion therapy encompass those seeking support for energy metabolism, cognitive function, and overall health. It may be particularly beneficial for individuals with conditions such as addiction, chronic fatigue syndrome, or neurodegenerative disorders. NAD+ can be combined with glutathione in IV therapy, providing added benefits in conditions like Parkinson's disease, chronic fatigue syndrome, and fibromyalgia.

The frequency of NAD+ infusion therapy depends on individual needs and responses to treatment, with some benefiting from weekly or bi-weekly infusions. Proper storage precautions, such as protection from light and an oxygen-free environment, are vital to maintain NAD+'s potency and efficacy.

While NAD+ infusion therapy shows promising results in improving energy metabolism, cognitive function, and overall health, further research is essential to establish optimal dosages, duration, and frequency for various health conditions. The book serves as an invaluable resource for healthcare professionals and individuals seeking comprehensive insights into the transformative potential of NAD+ infusion therapy.

Lipoic Acid

Lipoic acid and its biologically active form, alpha-lipoic acid (ALA), are often used interchangeably to describe the same compound. ALA serves as a coenzyme in glucose breakdown for energy production and ATP synthesis, the primary cellular energy source. Additionally, ALA acts as a potent antioxidant, neutralizing free radicals that contribute to oxidative damage and various diseases. While the body can synthesize ALA, supplementation has demonstrated health benefits, particularly in metabolic health and oxidative stress.

This book extensively explores the benefits of ALA, ranging from improved glucose metabolism and enhanced insulin sensitivity to reduced inflammation and bolstered antioxidant defense. ALA has shown promise in neuroprotection, with studies investigating its therapeutic potential in various neurological disorders.

Dosage recommendations for IV ALA administration depend on individual needs and specific health conditions, typically ranging from 300 to 600 mg per infusion. The frequency and duration of ALA infusions vary based on individual responses and needs.

ALA infusion therapy has been employed to treat diverse health conditions, including diabetic neuropathy, metabolic syndrome, hepatitis C, and neurodegenerative disorders such as Alzheimer's and Parkinson's disease. It has also been studied for potential therapeutic benefits in cardiovascular disease and cancer.

Despite ALA not being considered an essential nutrient due to endogenous production, signs of deficiency are not specific. However, individuals with certain health conditions, such as liver disease or diabetes, may exhibit lower ALA levels. Rare instances of ALA toxicity may manifest as gastrointestinal disturbances, skin rash, and, in individuals with diabetes, hypoglycemia. Anaphylactic reactions, though rare, can occur during IV ALA infusion, presenting severe allergic responses.

Contraindications include a history of thiamine deficiency, and it is not recommended for pregnant or breastfeeding women. Ideal candidates for ALA infusion include those seeking support for metabolic health, oxidative stress, and neurological function. ALA infusion therapy is often combined with other compounds, such as amino acids, vitamins, and minerals, to promote overall health and wellness. Treatment frequency varies, with some individuals benefiting from weekly or bi-weekly infusions.

Clinical information delves into the forms of ALA, daily dosage limits, storage instructions, preparation for IV infusion, and treatment protocols. The book emphasizes the importance of proper storage to ensure the efficacy of ALA supplements.

In conclusion, this comprehensive guide provides a nuanced understanding of alpha-lipoic acid, offering valuable insights for healthcare professionals, patients, and those interested in alternative treatments. By exploring the transformative potential of ALA infusion therapy, readers can make informed decisions to optimize health and well-being.

CHAPTER EIGHT
ESSENTIAL NUTRIENT LIKE COMPOUND

Chlorine

Choline, an indispensable nutrient, assumes a pivotal role in various physiological processes, encompassing the integrity of cell membranes, neurotransmitter synthesis, fat metabolism, and the maintenance of liver function. As a precursor to the neurotransmitter acetylcholine, Choline significantly contributes to memory, muscle control, and mood regulation. The book expounds upon the myriad benefits of Choline, elucidating its positive impact on cognitive function, liver health, cardiovascular well-being, and the support it provides to the nervous system.

Dosage recommendations for Choline in IV hydration therapy are contingent upon individual factors such as age, sex, medical history, and overall health. The Adequate Intake (AI) for Choline for adults is established at 425 mg/day for women and 550 mg/day for men. However, therapeutic dosages in IV hydration may differ and should be determined by healthcare professionals based on patient-specific needs and treatment goals.

Choline supplementation in IV hydration therapy exhibits potential efficacy in treating various conditions, including cognitive decline, fatty liver disease, depression, anxiety, neurological disorders, and high homocysteine levels. The book sheds light on the rarity of Choline deficiency, its potential signs, and the even rarer instances of toxicity, emphasizing the importance of a nuanced and personalized approach to its administration.

Contraindications for Choline infusion are discussed, particularly in individuals with specific medical conditions or those taking certain medications. The book underscores the need for caution in individuals with trimethylaminuria (TMAU), bipolar disorder, or a history of mania, as well as those with kidney or liver disease. A healthcare professional's careful monitoring of choline intake is deemed essential in cases of impaired kidney or liver function.

Ideal candidates for Choline infusion include individuals with choline deficiency, cognitive decline, liver dysfunction, or high homocysteine levels, with the caveat that a healthcare professional thoroughly assess each patient's unique needs and medical history to determine the appropriateness of Choline infusion.

The book also explores the coadministration of Choline with other compounds in IV hydration therapy, highlighting its inclusion in formulations like the "Myers' Cocktail" to provide comprehensive support.

The frequency of Choline IV treatments is discussed, emphasizing its variability based on patient-specific needs, the severity of the deficiency or condition being treated, and the recommendations of healthcare providers.

Special notes touch upon Choline's role in weight loss infusions, specifically the "MIC" (Methionine, Inositol, and Choline) cocktail, clarifying that this combination is typically administered as an intramuscular (IM) injection, not intravenous (IV), and should be complemented with a balanced diet and regular exercise for optimal results.

Clinical information on Choline covers its various forms, daily dosage limits, storage considerations, preparation for IV infusion, treatment protocols, half-life considerations, and stability, providing healthcare professionals and readers with a comprehensive understanding of this essential nutrient's intricacies.

Inositol

Inositol, also known as myo-inositol, is a naturally occurring sugar alcohol present in various foods such as fruits, beans, grains, and nuts. Its significance in cellular signaling and involvement in physiological processes, including insulin sensitivity, neurotransmitter modulation, and lipid metabolism, underscores its relevance in maintaining overall health. This comprehensive exploration delves into the multifaceted benefits of inositol.

Among its main advantages, inositol has demonstrated efficacy in mood regulation by positively influencing serotonin and dopamine receptors, potentially alleviating symptoms of anxiety and depression. Furthermore, its association with improved insulin sensitivity positions inositol as a potential asset for individuals with insulin resistance or type 2 diabetes. Studies also suggest its potential in managing Polycystic Ovary Syndrome (PCOS) by enhancing hormonal balance and metabolic markers, with additional benefits extending to fertility-related concerns in women with PCOS. Inositol's impact on lipid metabolism contributes to maintaining healthy cholesterol levels and supporting liver function.

Determining the appropriate dosage for inositol in IV hydration therapy requires consideration of individual factors such as age, sex, medical history, and overall health. While no established daily intake exists, oral supplementation typically ranges from 500 mg to 18 g per day, with the therapeutic dosage for IV inositol varying based on specific patient needs and treatment goals.

Conditions that may benefit from inositol supplementation in IV hydration therapy include mood disorders, insulin resistance, PCOS, fertility issues related to PCOS, high cholesterol levels, or fatty liver disease. While inositol deficiency is rare due to its synthesis by the body and dietary sources, signs may manifest as mood disturbances, insulin resistance, PCOS symptoms, and fertility issues.

Inositol toxicity is uncommon, but excessive intake may result in gastrointestinal issues, dizziness, or fatigue. Contraindications exist for individuals taking antidepressants, lithium, antipsychotic medications, or anti-anxiety medications, requiring caution and consultation with healthcare providers.

Ideal candidates for inositol infusion encompass individuals with mood disorders, insulin resistance, PCOS, fertility issues, or lipid metabolism problems. However, a thorough assessment by a healthcare professional is crucial to determine the appropriateness of inositol infusion for each patient.

The book explores the coadministration of inositol with other compounds in IV hydration therapy, emphasizing its integration into nutrient infusion formulas like the "Myers' Cocktail." The frequency of inositol IV treatments varies based on patient needs, the severity of the deficiency or condition, and healthcare provider recommendations, ranging from weekly to monthly.

Special notes highlight inositol's role in weight loss infusions, such as the "MIC" cocktail, emphasizing the importance of a balanced diet and regular exercise for optimal results.

Clinical information covers various aspects, including inositol's forms, daily dosage limits, storage instructions, preparation for IV infusion, treatment protocols, half-life considerations, and stability. This comprehensive guide serves as an invaluable resource for healthcare professionals and individuals seeking to understand and harness the potential benefits of inositol in IV hydration therapy.

Nutrient Like Compounds

In addition to compounds utilized in intravenous (IV) therapy, there exists a category of essential nutrients not directly employed in this method but pivotal for overall health and well-being. A comprehensive understanding of these compounds is instrumental as they can serve as valuable supplements between IV therapy sessions. Among these compounds, phytochemicals take precedence, representing naturally occurring substances found in plants. Prominent examples include carotenoids, flavonoids, and resveratrol, each renowned for possessing antioxidant and anti-inflammatory properties.

Phytochemicals

Phytochemicals play a crucial role in safeguarding against chronic diseases such as cancer and heart disease. The most advantageous sources of these compounds are diverse arrays of whole, unprocessed plant-based foods. These include fruits, vegetables, whole grains, legumes, nuts, seeds, herbs, and spices. Notable examples of phytochemical-rich food sources include berries (e.g., blueberries, strawberries, raspberries, blackberries) teeming with anthocyanins and flavonoids, and cruciferous vegetables (e.g., broccoli, cauliflower, kale, Brussels sprouts) containing sulforaphane, indoles, and isothiocyanates.

Tomatoes emerge as a noteworthy source of lycopene, while leafy greens (e.g., spinach, collard greens, Swiss chard) contribute carotenoids, lutein, and zeaxanthin. Grapes and red wine boast resveratrol and other polyphenols, while citrus fruits (e.g., oranges, lemons, grapefruits) contain flavonoids like hesperidin and naringenin. Green tea proves valuable with its catechins, notably epigallocatechin-3-gallate (EGCG), and dark chocolate and cocoa are rich in flavanols and other polyphenols. Legumes (e.g., beans, lentils, chickpeas) encompass various phytochemicals, including isoflavones, phytic acid, and saponins, while nuts and seeds (e.g., walnuts, flaxseeds, chia seeds) provide lignans and additional phytochemicals. Lastly, herbs and spices (e.g., turmeric, ginger, cinnamon, rosemary) encompass a diverse spectrum of phytochemicals, including curcumin, gingerol, and cinnamaldehyde.

To optimize the health benefits of phytochemicals, it is advised to embrace a dietary regimen incorporating a diverse and colorful spectrum of plant-based foods. The varying hues and types of foods not only enhance culinary experiences but also offer an assortment of phytochemicals, each endowed with unique health-promoting properties.

In essence, the inclusion of a wide variety of fruits, vegetables, whole grains, legumes, nuts, seeds, herbs, and spices in one's diet ensures a robust intake of these invaluable compounds, fostering overall health and well-being.

Fiber

Fiber, while not classified as a nutrient, holds a pivotal role in promoting optimal digestive health. It is a type of carbohydrate that remains indigestible by the body, yet its contributions to overall well-being are substantial. One of its primary functions lies in the regulation of digestion and bowel movements, and it is also recognized for potential benefits such as lowering cholesterol and blood sugar levels.

The most beneficial sources of fiber are derived from plant-based foods, encompassing a diverse array of whole grains, fruits, vegetables, legumes, nuts, and seeds. Whole grains such as whole wheat, brown rice, quinoa, barley, oats, and bulgur stand out for their richness in fiber content. Opting for whole-grain variants of bread, pasta, and cereals becomes a strategic choice to enhance daily fiber intake.

Fruits offer a delectable and nutritious means of incorporating fiber into one's diet, with options like raspberries, blackberries, pears, apples (particularly with the skin intact), oranges, and bananas serving as excellent sources. A varied selection of fruits ensures a balanced intake of both soluble and insoluble fibers, each contributing distinct advantages to digestive health.

The inclusion of an assortment of vegetables further augments fiber intake, with leafy greens, broccoli, cauliflower, Brussels sprouts, sweet potatoes, carrots, and artichokes being particularly fiber-rich choices. This diversity not only enhances the nutritional profile of meals but also provides a spectrum of fibers for comprehensive digestive support.

Legumes, including beans (such as black beans, kidney beans, pinto beans, and white beans), lentils, and chickpeas, emerge as formidable contenders in the realm of fiber-rich foods. Their versatility allows for seamless integration into various dishes such as salads, soups, and stews, presenting an easy and flavorful means of incorporating additional fiber into the diet.

Nuts and seeds, including almonds, pistachios, chia seeds, flaxseeds, and sunflower seeds, contribute not only to dietary fiber but also to a range of essential nutrients. These can be savored as snacks, integrated into salads, or used as toppings for yogurt or oatmeal, providing a satisfying and wholesome method of boosting fiber intake.

For those seeking to supplement their fiber intake, psyllium husk serves as a natural and effective dietary fiber supplement derived from the seed husks of the Plantago ovata plant. This versatile supplement can be seamlessly incorporated into various foods, including smoothies, oatmeal, or yogurt, offering an additional avenue to elevate overall fiber consumption.

In summary, while not classified as a nutrient, fiber plays a vital role in supporting digestive health. By incorporating a diverse array of plant-based foods rich in fiber, individuals can not only ensure optimal digestive function but also reap the additional benefits associated with enhanced overall well-being.

Probiotics

Probiotics, classified as live microorganisms, predominantly encompassing bacteria and yeasts, confer a spectrum of health benefits when ingested in sufficient quantities. Their pivotal roles include the maintenance of a harmonious balance in gut bacteria, facilitation of digestion, and augmentation of immune function. The most effective sources of probiotics are derived from fermented foods, wherein the fermentation process fosters the proliferation of beneficial microorganisms.

A myriad of exemplary probiotic-rich foods exists, each contributing unique strains to fortify gut health. Among these, yogurt stands out as one of the most widely recognized probiotic foods. Formulated by fermenting milk with specific bacteria, such as Lactobacillus and Bifidobacterium strains, quality yogurt bears the label "live and active cultures," denoting the presence of probiotics.

Kefir, a fermented milk drink akin to yogurt but with a thinner consistency, is crafted by fermenting milk with a blend of bacteria and yeasts known as kefir grains. Notably, kefir often encompasses a broader array of probiotics compared to yogurt.

Sauerkraut, a product of fermented cabbage, particularly rich in Lactobacillus strains, is a noteworthy probiotic source. It is imperative to select unpasteurized sauerkraut to ensure the preservation of beneficial bacteria, as pasteurization can compromise their viability.

Kimchi, a traditional Korean dish comprising fermented vegetables, predominantly cabbage, seasoned with an array of spices, offers a robust source of probiotics, including Lactobacillus and other beneficial bacteria.

Tempeh, a fermented soybean product renowned as a plant-based protein source, boasts high probiotic content, specifically the Rhizopus oligosporus strain.

Miso, a traditional Japanese seasoning derived from fermented soybeans, is replete with probiotics, incorporating Lactobacillus and Bifidobacterium strains. It finds common use in soups and sauces.

Kombucha, a fermented tea beverage, encompasses a blend of bacteria and yeasts, delivering probiotic advantages. Available in various flavors, kombucha is gaining popularity as a probiotic-rich beverage.

Fermented pickles, immersed in a saltwater brine, offer a commendable source of Lactobacillus bacteria. It is important to note that pickles made with vinegar lack live probiotics.

Traditional buttermilk, the residual liquid post-butter churning, is a historical source of probiotics. However, it is pertinent to recognize that commercially available buttermilk is often cultured, with bacteria added to milk, potentially differing in probiotic benefits from its traditional counterpart.

Incorporating a diverse array of these fermented foods into one's diet ensures a comprehensive and ample intake of probiotics, contributing substantively to the support of gut health. While probiotic supplements are available, seeking guidance from a healthcare provider before initiating any supplementation is imperative. This holistic approach to integrating probiotics into one's dietary regimen underscores the importance of informed decision-making for optimal health and well-being.

Prebiotics

Prebiotics, integral components of a gut-friendly diet, are non-digestible fibers that act as nourishment for probiotics—beneficial bacteria residing in the gastrointestinal tract. This symbiotic relationship plays a pivotal role in supporting digestive health and contributing to overall well-being. Among the key sources of prebiotics are plant-based foods renowned for their richness in specific types of fibers, notably inulin, oligofructose, and galacto-oligosaccharides (GOS).

Chicory root, recognized as one of the richest sources of inulin, stands out as a versatile ingredient, serving as a coffee substitute or enhancing various recipes to elevate fiber intake. Jerusalem artichokes, also known as sunchokes, offer a tuberous source high in inulin and can be savored raw, cooked, or roasted. Dandelion greens, abundant in prebiotic fibers, add nutritional value to salads, soups, or as a sautéed side dish. Garlic, with its inulin content, not only imparts flavor to diverse dishes but also contributes to gut health. Onions, whether consumed raw or cooked, offer prebiotic fibers such as inulin and oligofructose. Leeks, akin to onions, present a rich source of prebiotic fibers, complementing soups, stews, and other culinary creations. Asparagus, known for its versatility, serves as a good source of inulin and can be prepared through steaming, grilling, or roasting.

Bananas, particularly unripe (green) ones, emerge as a valuable prebiotic source due to their high resistant starch content. Whole grains, encompassing barley, oats, and whole wheat, contribute prebiotic fibers like beta-glucan and oligosaccharides, fostering the growth of beneficial gut bacteria. Legumes, including beans, lentils, and chickpeas, stand out as rich sources of both prebiotic fibers and resistant starch, making them excellent additions to a gut-friendly diet.

Incorporating a diverse array of these prebiotic-rich foods into one's diet serves as an effective strategy to nurture the growth and activity of beneficial gut bacteria, thereby promoting optimal digestive health. The synergistic effect achieved by combining prebiotic-rich foods with probiotic-rich foods or supplements further enhances the overall benefits for a thriving gut ecosystem. This strategic dietary approach not only supports digestive health but also underscores the intricate interplay between nutrition and the intricate microbial communities within our gastrointestinal tract.

Omega-3 Fatty Acids

Omega-3 fatty acids, a subtype of polyunsaturated fats, hold paramount significance in promoting optimal brain and heart health while exhibiting potential anti-inflammatory properties, thereby mitigating the risk of chronic diseases. This category encompasses essential nutrients, namely eicosapentaenoic acid (EPA), docosahexaenoic acid (DHA), and alpha-linolenic acid (ALA), each playing pivotal roles in sustaining cardiovascular well-being, facilitating cognitive functions, and curbing inflammation within the body.

The diverse spectrum of omega-3 fatty acids finds its most abundant sources in specific dietary components. Fatty fish, including salmon, mackerel, sardines, anchovies, herring, and trout, emerge as rich reservoirs of EPA and DHA. Recommendations advocate a minimum consumption of two servings of fatty fish weekly to ensure a robust intake of these essential fatty acids.

Supplements derived from fish oil, sourced from species like cod, salmon, or krill, represent an alternative avenue for obtaining EPA and DHA. Particularly beneficial for individuals with infrequent fish consumption or challenges in meeting omega-3 needs through dietary means, these supplements provide a convenient and concentrated source of these essential fatty acids.

For those adhering to plant-based dietary preferences, algae oil supplements offer a suitable solution, as microalgae serve as primary producers of DHA in the marine food chain. This alternative ensures the acquisition of DHA without the reliance on fish or fish oil, making it an ideal choice for vegans and vegetarians.

Plant-based sources of alpha-linolenic acid (ALA), a precursor to EPA and DHA, include nutrient-dense seeds such as chia seeds, flaxseeds, and hemp seeds. Walnuts, among nuts, stand out as a valuable source of plant-based omega-3 fatty acids, particularly ALA. Additionally, certain plant oils like flaxseed oil, canola oil, and soybean oil contribute to ALA intake.

It is crucial to acknowledge that the conversion of ALA to EPA and DHA within the human body is relatively inefficient. Consequently, while plant-based omega-3 sources may not confer identical benefits as those derived from fatty fish, incorporating a variety of plant-based ALA sources can still bolster overall omega-3 intake, offering health benefits, especially pertinent to vegetarians and vegans.

To ensure a comprehensive and sufficient intake of omega-3 fatty acids, a balanced approach is recommended. This entails integrating a combination of fatty fish, plant-based ALA sources, or, when necessary, high-quality supplements into one's dietary regimen. Such a multifaceted strategy not only accommodates diverse dietary preferences but also aligns with the overarching goal of promoting holistic health through omega-3 fatty acid enrichment.

CHAPTER NINE
PEPTIDES

Disclaimer: The utilization of peptides in medical and research contexts is subject to stringent regulations. In the United States, the Food and Drug Administration (FDA) oversees the use of peptides as pharmaceuticals, while research applications are governed by regulations set forth by esteemed organizations like the National Institutes of Health (NIH) and the International Council for Harmonisation of Technical Requirements for Pharmaceuticals for Human Use (ICH). These regulatory bodies establish standards for the safety and efficacy of peptides, overseeing their utilization in clinical trials and approved medical treatments. It is crucial to recognize that the deployment of peptides for non-medical purposes, such as in sports performance enhancement or cosmetic treatments, may lack comparable regulatory oversight, potentially posing additional risks. The information presented in this chapter is intended solely for educational purposes. Any protocols devised should receive approval from a medical director and prioritize the well-being of clients.

Peptides, composed of short chains of amino acids, exhibit diverse biological functions within the human body. While amino acids serve as the fundamental building blocks of proteins, peptides possess unique structures and functions that can contribute to health and wellness. Their distinct structure facilitates easy absorption and utilization due to their small size and specific amino acid sequences, rendering them more stable than free amino acids that are prone to rapid breakdown in the body. Furthermore, peptides can be tailored to target specific biological processes, potentially enhancing their effectiveness in delivering health benefits. The following elucidates the reasons why peptides may be preferred over amino acids for health and wellness:

1. **Specificity:** Peptides can be customized to target precise biological processes, such as stimulating collagen production for improved skin health and wrinkle reduction.

2. **Bioavailability:** Due to their small size and structure, peptides can be efficiently absorbed and utilized by the body, enhancing their effectiveness in delivering targeted health benefits.

3. **Stability:** Peptides demonstrate greater stability compared to free amino acids, ensuring a sustained delivery of intended health benefits over time.

4. **Safety:** Generally deemed safe for human consumption as naturally occurring compounds, peptides warrant consultation with a healthcare professional before use for health and wellness purposes, in line with any supplement.

The unique structural features of peptides make them valuable contributors to health and wellness. Certain peptides have been studied for their potential effects on muscle growth, weight loss, anti-aging, and overall health. Notable peptides in health and wellness include:

- **BPC-157:** Known as "Body Protective Compound," it has demonstrated potential in wound healing, tissue repair, and reducing inflammation.

- **Ipamorelin:** A growth hormone-releasing peptide (GHRP) studied for promoting muscle growth, fat loss, and overall body composition improvement.

- **CJC-1295:** A growth hormone-releasing hormone (GHRH) analog, often used with Ipamorelin, to stimulate growth hormone release, potentially promoting muscle growth, fat loss, and improved recovery.

- **Thymosin Beta-4 (TB-500):** Explored for its potential in wound healing, tissue repair, and anti-inflammatory effects.

- **Thymosin Alpha-1:** Known for boosting the immune system, with potential applications in treating chronic viral and immunodeficiency diseases.

- **GHK-Cu (Copper Peptide):** Recognized for skin rejuvenation, wound healing, and anti-inflammatory properties in skincare products.

- **Growth hormone-releasing hormone (GHRH) analogs:** Utilized to stimulate growth hormone release for athletic performance enhancement and anti-aging effects.

- **Melanotan II:** Stimulates melanin production for tanning and skin protection purposes, typically administered via subcutaneous injection.

- **Cerebrolysin:** Used for neurological purposes such as improving cognitive function, treating Alzheimer's disease, and stroke.

- **GLP-1 (Semaglutide):** A naturally occurring peptide hormone used as a medication to treat type 2 diabetes and obesity, administered by injection.

In some cases, peptides are incorporated into IV hydration, particularly in anti-aging or regenerative medicine. However, the safety and efficacy of this approach are yet to be firmly established, warranting further research. Some peptides, such as BPC-157, are studied for potential benefits in promoting healing and tissue regeneration in IV hydration. Peptides like CJC-1295 and Ipamorelin may be used in IV hydration for their potential to stimulate growth hormone release and promote muscle growth. Nevertheless, consulting with a healthcare professional before employing peptides in IV hydration or any medical context is imperative.

While certain peptides are available in oral form, it's essential to acknowledge that the bioavailability of oral peptides may be limited due to susceptibility to enzymatic degradation in the digestive tract. Consequently, oral peptides may not match the efficacy of injections or infusions.

In the realm of dietary supplementation, a variety of oral peptide supplements are currently accessible in the market, with notable examples including collagen peptides and select nootropic peptides. These supplements are meticulously designed, often incorporating advanced strategies to enhance stability and bioavailability, such as encapsulation or conjugation with protective molecules.

Collagen peptides, derived from hydrolyzed collagen found in connective tissues like skin, bones, and cartilage, are particularly noteworthy. Formulated as powders or capsules, they can be ingested orally or applied topically. The primary applications of collagen peptides revolve around promoting skin health, mitigating signs of aging, and supporting joint functionality. The availability of oral collagen supplements for promoting skin health, reducing wrinkles, and enhancing joint function is complemented by the utilization of topical collagen creams and serums for similar purposes.

While there is currently no intravenous (IV) form of collagen peptides, other IV infusions, such as those containing vitamin C and amino acids, have demonstrated potential in promoting collagen production. These infusions are harnessed for diverse health and wellness objectives, including the enhancement of skin health and the reduction of aging indicators.

Another category of oral peptides gaining prominence is that of nootropic peptides, renowned for their purported cognitive-enhancing properties. These peptides are believed to foster mental acuity, memory retention, and concentration, making them sought-after supplements for supporting cognitive health and function. Noteworthy examples in this category include Semax, derived from the adrenocorticotropic hormone (ACTH), with purported benefits in enhancing cognitive function and alleviating anxiety. Additionally, Selank, a synthetic peptide, is thought to exhibit anxiolytic and nootropic effects, offering potential stress reduction and relaxation promotion. Lastly, Noopept, another synthetic peptide, is believed to enhance memory, learning, and attention span, presenting potential benefits in supporting cognitive function and preventing cognitive decline.

BPC -157

BPC-157, or Body Protection Compound-157, is a synthetic peptide comprised of 15 amino acids. This peptide has garnered attention due to its potential therapeutic and regenerative properties within the human body. Originating from a segment of the protein found in human gastric juice, BPC-157 is believed to elicit the production of growth factors, fostering tissue repair and regeneration. The specific amino acids constituting BPC-157 include Glycine (x2), L-Proline (x4), L-Arginine, L-Lysine, L-Alanine, L-Aspartic Acid, L-Serine, L-Glutamic Acid, L-Leucine, L-Valine, and L-Threonine.

Unlike naturally occurring peptides, BPC-157 is a product of chemical synthesis and is not indigenous to the human body. It is primarily available for research purposes, facilitating scientific and medical investigations. Numerous studies have explored the potential therapeutic benefits of BPC-157, which include its capacity to promote wound healing, diminish inflammation, enhance tissue repair, and improve joint function.

The peptide's mechanisms of action are believed to involve the stimulation of growth factor production and the promotion of angiogenesis, the formation of new blood vessels. Consequently, increased blood flow and oxygenation to affected tissues may contribute to heightened healing and regeneration. Additionally, BPC-157 exhibits anti-inflammatory effects, potentially alleviating pain associated with various medical conditions.

For intravenous infusion, the recommended daily dosage of BPC-157 typically ranges from 250-1000 mcg, although individual needs and health status may influence dosages. Administration typically occurs once a day, and the duration of treatment varies based on the specific medical condition and the individual's response to the peptide.

BPC-157 has demonstrated therapeutic potential in diverse medical conditions, such as wound healing, tissue repair in muscles and tendons, joint function enhancement, ulcerative colitis, traumatic brain injury, and spinal cord injury. Although signs of BPC-157 deficiency are unknown due to its synthetic nature, the peptide has exhibited a favorable safety profile in human studies, with potential side effects including gastrointestinal disturbances, headaches, and dizziness.

Contraindications for BPC-157 include hypersensitivity to any of its components. Individuals seeking BPC-157 infusion to enhance healing and recovery, especially in cases of injuries or conditions affecting tissue repair, should consult with a qualified healthcare professional to assess its appropriateness. The frequency of treatments is individualized based on specific needs and health status.

BPC-157 is available in lyophilized powder form for reconstitution in sterile water or saline solution. The daily dosage limits and optimal treatment protocols for different medical conditions remain areas of ongoing research. Proper storage involves keeping BPC-157 at room temperature or below, protected from light. The peptide is typically reconstituted in sterile water or saline solution before administration, commonly through intravenous, intramuscular, or subcutaneous routes. The half-life and stability of BPC-157 necessitate further research to establish its pharmacokinetic properties definitively.

Ipamorelin

Ipamorelin, a synthetic peptide classified as a growth hormone secretagogue, is a compound comprising five amino acids—alanine, glycine, histidine, lysine, and tryptophan. It has garnered attention for its potential impact on augmenting growth hormone secretion and positively influencing body composition. Unlike naturally occurring peptides, Ipamorelin is produced through chemical synthesis and is accessible as a research chemical, primarily intended for scientific and medical research applications.

Research into Ipamorelin suggests a spectrum of therapeutic benefits, including heightened growth hormone secretion, improved body composition, enhanced bone density, and a potential reduction in the risk of age-related diseases. Its versatility extends to potential applications in treating conditions such as growth hormone deficiency, osteoporosis, and sarcopenia. The primary mechanism of action involves stimulating growth hormone release from the pituitary gland, leading to elevated growth hormone levels, potentially resulting in improved body composition, enhanced bone density, and a decreased risk of age-related ailments.

Noteworthy is Ipamorelin's favorable safety profile, believed to exhibit fewer side effects compared to other growth hormone secretagogues. For intravenous infusion, the recommended daily dosage typically ranges between 200-300 mcg, subject to individual health status and needs. However, the safety and efficacy of different dosages and treatment durations remain areas necessitating further research to establish optimal protocols for varying medical conditions.

Ipamorelin has been explored for potential therapeutic applications in conditions such as growth hormone deficiency, osteoporosis, and sarcopenia. Its use may be particularly relevant for individuals seeking to enhance body composition, improve bone density, and mitigate age-related disease risks. To determine suitability, consultation with a qualified healthcare professional is crucial.

The frequency of Ipamorelin infusion varies based on individual needs and health status, necessitating personalized treatment plans under the guidance of healthcare professionals. Clinical studies involving animals and humans have indicated its potential therapeutic benefits in stimulating growth hormone release and improving body composition.

Ipamorelin is available in lyophilized powder form for reconstitution in sterile water or saline solution. Despite its increasing usage, the daily dosage limits remain undetermined, requiring further research for different medical conditions. Proper storage of Ipamorelin involves room temperature or below and protection from light. Preparation for intravenous infusion involves reconstitution in sterile water or saline solution, with administration typically intravenous but also potentially subcutaneous. The optimal treatment protocols, including dosages, durations, and frequency, require additional research to establish their efficacy for diverse medical conditions.

The half-life of Ipamorelin is approximately 2 hours, and when stored correctly, it is considered stable at room temperature or below and protected from light. These factors collectively contribute to the evolving understanding and utilization of Ipamorelin in scientific and medical research contexts.

CJC-1295

CJC-1295, a synthetic peptide classified under growth hormone-releasing hormones (GHRHs), consists of 29 amino acids. Investigated for its potential impact on growth hormone secretion and body composition enhancement, its amino acid sequence is delineated as Tyr-D-Ala-Asp-Ala-Ile-Phe-Thr-Gln-Ser-Tyr-Arg-Lys-Val-Leu-Ala-Gln-Leu-Ser-Ala-Arg-Lys-Leu-Leu-Gln-Asp-Ile-Leu-Ser-Arg-NH2.

This synthetic peptide is not endogenously present in the human body; instead, it is chemically synthesized and utilized as a research chemical for scientific and medical investigations. CJC-1295 has garnered attention for its therapeutic potential, including fostering growth hormone secretion, augmenting body composition, improving bone density, and mitigating age-related diseases. It may hold promise in addressing conditions such as growth hormone deficiency, osteoporosis, and sarcopenia.

The primary mechanism of CJC-1295 is believed to involve stimulating growth hormone release from the pituitary gland, resulting in increased growth hormone levels. Notably, it exhibits a favorable safety profile with potentially fewer side effects compared to other growth hormone-releasing peptides.

Dosage recommendations typically range between 1-2 mg per week for intravenous infusion, administered once or twice weekly. However, optimal dosages and treatment durations remain undetermined, necessitating further research to establish guidelines for various medical conditions.

CJC-1295 has been explored for therapeutic applications in growth hormone deficiency, osteoporosis, and sarcopenia. No signs of CJC-1295 deficiency are identified, given its synthetic nature. While generally safe, potential side effects may include headache, flushing, and nausea. Contraindications involve hypersensitivity to its components.

Ideal candidates for CJC-1295 infusion are individuals seeking improvements in body composition, bone density, and age-related disease risk reduction. The frequency of treatments varies based on individual needs, requiring consultation with a qualified healthcare professional.

Available as a lyophilized powder, CJC-1295 is reconstituted in sterile water or saline solution for intravenous administration. Storage is recommended at room temperature or below, shielded from light. Treatment protocols, optimal dosages, and treatment durations remain subjects of ongoing research, as does determining the daily dosage limit for various medical conditions.

The half-life of CJC-1295 is approximately 7-8 days, rendering it stable under proper storage conditions. Its stability underscores its potential utility in scientific and medical investigations, albeit with a need for continued research to refine treatment protocols and dosage parameters.

Thymosin Beta-4

Thymosin Beta-4 (Tβ4) is a small peptide composed of 43 amino acids that naturally occurs in the human body, playing a pivotal role in diverse biological processes, including cell differentiation, tissue repair, and angiogenesis. The peptide is present in various tissues and cells, such as platelets, endothelial cells, and white blood cells.

Thymosin Beta-4 has garnered attention for its potential therapeutic benefits, encompassing tissue repair promotion, inflammation reduction, and accelerated wound healing. Its applications in medical conditions like skin ulcers, myocardial infarction, and spinal cord injury are currently under investigation. The proposed mechanisms of action include the facilitation of cell migration and differentiation crucial for tissue repair and regeneration, along with potential anti-inflammatory and antioxidative effects.

Recommended dosages typically range between 1.6 and 2.0 mg per day, administered via intravenous infusion over several weeks to months, once or twice a week. Nevertheless, the optimal dosage and treatment duration remain undetermined, necessitating further research to establish precise protocols for varying medical conditions.

Thymosin Beta-4 shows promise in treating skin ulcers, myocardial infarction, and spinal cord injuries, although its deficiency signs are unknown due to its naturally occurring nature. The peptide exhibits a favorable safety profile, with potential side effects such as headache, flushing, and nausea.

While generally considered safe, Thymosin Beta-4 is contraindicated in individuals with hypersensitivity to its components. Potential candidates for Thymosin Beta-4 infusion include those seeking enhanced tissue repair, reduced inflammation, and improved wound healing. The frequency of treatments varies based on individual needs and health status, necessitating consultation with a qualified healthcare professional.

Clinical studies involving animals and humans support Thymosin Beta-4's therapeutic potential, demonstrating its efficacy in promoting tissue repair, reducing inflammation, and accelerating wound healing. The peptide is versatile in administration, including intravenous and subcutaneous injections or topical application.

As for storage, Thymosin Beta-4 should be stored at room temperature or below, shielded from light. Preparation for intravenous infusion involves reconstitution in sterile water or saline solution. However, treatment protocols, optimal dosages, and the half-life of Thymosin Beta-4 require further investigation for comprehensive understanding and application in clinical settings.

Thymosin Alpha-1

Thymosin Alpha-1 (Tα1) is a bioactive peptide composed of 28 amino acids that occurs naturally in the human body. Its presence is noted in various tissues and cells, including the thymus gland, spleen, and lymph nodes. Functionally, Thymosin Alpha-1 plays a crucial role in modulating immune responses and orchestrating anti-inflammatory processes.

Extensive research has explored the therapeutic potential of Thymosin Alpha-1, revealing its capacity to enhance immune functions, mitigate inflammation, and facilitate tissue repair. This peptide exhibits promising applications in addressing diverse medical conditions, such as viral infections (e.g., hepatitis B and C, HIV), cancer, and autoimmune disorders like rheumatoid arthritis.

Dosage recommendations for Thymosin Alpha-1 typically involve intravenous infusion, with suggested weekly doses ranging from 1.6 to 3.2 mg. However, individual variations and health status may influence specific dosage requirements, and the frequency of administration can be adjusted accordingly. It is imperative to note that optimal dosages and treatment durations are yet to be firmly established, necessitating further research to refine protocols for different medical conditions.

Thymosin Alpha-1 has shown a favorable safety profile, with documented tolerability in human studies. Noteworthy side effects may include headache, fatigue, and localized reactions at the injection site. While generally considered safe, caution is warranted for individuals with hypersensitivity to any of its components.

Suitable candidates for Thymosin Alpha-1 infusion are those seeking to bolster immune function, regulate inflammation, and facilitate tissue repair. Determining the most suitable treatment plan requires consultation with a qualified healthcare professional.

The frequency of Thymosin Alpha-1 treatments varies based on individual needs and health status, typically administered once or twice a week over several weeks to months. Clinical investigations in both animal and human studies have substantiated its efficacy in enhancing immune responses, mitigating inflammation, and promoting tissue repair.

Thymosin Alpha-1 is commercially available as a lyophilized powder for reconstitution in sterile water or saline solution. However, daily dosage limits have not been definitively established, underscoring the need for further research to delineate optimal dosages for specific medical conditions.

Proper storage conditions mandate room temperature or below, shielding from light. Prior to intravenous infusion, Thymosin Alpha-1 should be reconstituted in sterile water or saline solution. The half-life of Thymosin Alpha-1 is approximately 2 hours, and it remains stable under proper storage conditions.

In summary, Thymosin Alpha-1 holds considerable promise in the realm of therapeutic interventions, yet ongoing research is essential to refine dosage recommendations, treatment protocols, and its applications across diverse medical conditions.

GHK-Cu

GHK-Cu, also known as Copper Tripeptide-1, is a small peptide composed of three amino acids—glycine, histidine, and lysine—along with a copper ion. It naturally occurs within the human body and plays a crucial role in various biological processes, notably tissue repair and regeneration. This peptide is present in diverse tissues and cells, including blood, saliva, and urine.

Research on GHK-Cu has explored its potential therapeutic benefits, encompassing tissue repair promotion, inflammation reduction, and enhancement of antioxidant activity. The peptide may find applications in treating conditions such as skin aging, wound healing, and neurodegenerative disorders. Its mechanism of action is believed to involve stimulating collagen and elastin production, essential proteins for healthy skin and connective tissues. Additionally, GHK-Cu may possess anti-inflammatory properties and mitigate oxidative stress in damaged tissues.

Dosage recommendations for GHK-Cu infusion typically range between 1-2 mg per week, though individual requirements may vary. Administration frequency is usually once or twice a week, with treatment duration contingent on the individual's condition and response.

GHK-Cu has undergone scrutiny for its potential therapeutic applications in skin aging, wound healing, and neurodegenerative disorders, such as Alzheimer's disease. Although no signs of GHK-Cu deficiency are known, its safety profile appears favorable, with potential side effects including headache, fatigue, and injection site reactions.

While generally considered safe, GHK-Cu is contraindicated in individuals hypersensitive to its components. Eligible candidates for GHK-Cu infusion include those seeking tissue repair and regeneration, inflammation reduction, and enhanced antioxidant activity. Consultation with a qualified healthcare professional is crucial to determine an appropriate treatment plan.

The frequency of GHK-Cu treatments varies based on individual needs, typically administered once or twice a week over several weeks to months. Clinical studies have explored its therapeutic potential, but further research is necessary to establish optimal dosages and treatment protocols.

GHK-Cu is available in various forms, including lyophilized powder for reconstitution, topical creams, and serums. Daily dosage limits are yet to be well-established, and research is ongoing to determine optimal dosages for different medical conditions. Storage guidelines recommend room temperature or below and protection from light.

Preparation for GHK-Cu IV infusion involves reconstitution in sterile water or saline solution. The peptide is administered intravenously, with treatment protocols still under investigation. GHK-Cu has an approximate half-life of six hours and is generally stable when stored properly. Ongoing research aims to provide a more comprehensive understanding of its therapeutic applications and optimal usage guidelines.

Growth Hormone-Releasing Hormone

Growth hormone-releasing hormone (GHRH) is a peptide hormone intricately involved in the stimulation of growth hormone (GH) production and release from the pituitary gland. This natural peptide is synthesized in the hypothalamus of the brain, playing a vital role in various physiological processes, notably in the realms of growth and metabolism.

The production and release of GHRH occur in the hypothalamus, where it is then released into the bloodstream. Subsequently, it travels to the pituitary gland, where it exerts its influence on the synthesis and secretion of growth hormone. This intricate regulatory process underscores the significance of GHRH in orchestrating hormonal balance.

Scientific scrutiny of GHRH has revealed potential therapeutic benefits, extending to areas such as augmenting muscle mass and strength, enhancing bone density, mitigating body fat accumulation, and improving cognitive function. The exploration of its applications in medical conditions, such as growth hormone deficiency, osteoporosis, and age-related cognitive decline, adds further depth to its potential medical significance.

Dosage recommendations for GHRH, particularly when administered through intravenous (IV) infusion, typically range between 0.1-1 mcg/kg body weight per day. However, individualized dosages may be necessary based on specific health needs and conditions. The peptide is generally administered once or twice daily, and the treatment duration varies based on individual responses and conditions. It is crucial to note that the safety and efficacy of GHRH at different dosages and durations require further elucidation through ongoing research.

GHRH exhibits promise in the therapeutic landscape for addressing conditions such as growth hormone deficiency, osteoporosis, and age-related cognitive decline. Signs of GHRH deficiency include diminished muscle mass and strength, increased body fat, reduced bone density, and cognitive decline. Conversely, potential side effects or toxicity of GHRH may manifest as headache, nausea, vomiting, and injection site reactions.

While GHRH is generally considered safe for human use, like any medical intervention, potential risks and side effects exist. Contraindications involve individuals with hypersensitivity to any of its components. The candidacy for GHRH infusion is often determined by individuals seeking improvements in muscle mass, bone density, body fat reduction, and cognitive function, with guidance from qualified healthcare professionals.

The frequency of GHRH treatments varies based on individual needs and health status, typically administered once or twice daily over several weeks to months. Numerous clinical trials have been conducted to assess the safety and efficacy of GHRH, although ongoing research is imperative to refine dosages and treatment protocols for diverse medical conditions.

GHRH is available in various forms, including lyophilized powder for reconstitution in sterile water or saline solution, as well as in subcutaneous injection form. The absence of well-established daily dosage limits necessitates further research to determine optimal dosages for different medical conditions.

Proper storage of GHRH at room temperature or below, shielded from light, ensures its stability. Preparation for IV infusion involves reconstitution in sterile water or saline solution, with administration typically carried out intravenously. The half-life of GHRH is approximately 10-20 minutes, emphasizing the need for careful consideration in treatment protocols.

In conclusion, while GHRH holds promise in therapeutic applications, comprehensive research is imperative to define optimal dosages, treatment durations, and frequencies for various medical conditions.

Melanotan II

Melanotan II is a synthetic peptide hormone structurally analogous to alpha-melanocyte-stimulating hormone (α-MSH), designed to induce melanin production in the skin, thereby enhancing tanning and pigmentation. Unlike naturally occurring peptides, Melanotan II is not endogenously present in the human body.

This synthetic peptide has been subject to extensive research exploring potential therapeutic benefits, including heightened tanning and pigmentation, potential protection against UV-induced skin damage, and even appetite suppression leading to weight loss. The recommended intravenous infusion dosage typically ranges between 0.5-1 mg per day, although individual requirements and health conditions may necessitate variations. Administration frequency, duration, and safety across different dosages remain subjects for further investigation.

Melanotan II has exhibited promise in addressing various medical conditions, including skin pigmentation disorders like vitiligo, potential reduction in UV-induced skin damage, and weight loss through appetite suppression. However, the optimal dosages and treatment protocols for specific conditions have not been conclusively established, necessitating ongoing research.

While Melanotan II deficiency is not a recognized medical condition, potential signs of toxicity include nausea, vomiting, headaches, flushing, increased blood pressure, skin discoloration, hyperpigmentation, and freckling. Contraindications include hypersensitivity to components, a history of skin cancer or related conditions, and pregnancy or breastfeeding.

Appropriate candidates for Melanotan II infusion are individuals seeking increased tanning, reduced UV-induced skin damage, and potential appetite suppression with weight loss. Consultation with a qualified healthcare professional is crucial for devising an individualized treatment plan.

Melanotan II is available in various administration forms, such as injections, nasal sprays, and skin patches. For intravenous infusion, it is typically prepared as a sterile lyophilized powder reconstituted with sterile water or saline solution.

Daily dosage limits and storage conditions, including cool, dry places away from direct sunlight and moisture, are important considerations. Preparation for intravenous infusion should be conducted by a qualified healthcare professional according to established guidelines.

Treatment protocols may vary based on individual needs and health status, with typical administration occurring once or twice a day over several weeks to months. The half-life of Melanotan II is approximately 30-60 minutes, indicating rapid elimination from the body after administration. While relatively stable under normal storage conditions, degradation may occur over time if not stored properly.

Cerebrolysin

Cerebrolysin, an innovative neuropeptide solution, is derived from pig brain tissue and encompasses a complex composition of peptides, amino acids, and neurotrophic factors. Recognized for its neuroprotective and neurorestorative properties, this substance finds widespread application in the management of various neurological disorders. The manufacturing process involves intricate extraction and purification techniques.

Cerebrolysin's multifaceted benefits extend to neurological health and function. These include neuroprotection, shielding the brain against toxins and trauma; neurorestoration, promoting neuronal growth and repair; cognitive enhancement, improving memory, attention, and executive function; and mood improvement, with potential alleviation of depression and anxiety symptoms.

Administered through daily intravenous infusions, Cerebrolysin dosage recommendations vary based on factors such as age, weight, medical history, and the specific condition being treated, typically ranging from 5-30 mL per day. This therapeutic agent has demonstrated efficacy in addressing conditions such as stroke, traumatic brain injury, Alzheimer's disease, Parkinson's disease, multiple sclerosis, dementia, cognitive impairment, depression, and anxiety.

There are no established signs of Cerebrolysin deficiency as it is not naturally produced in the body. Although generally well-tolerated, potential signs of toxicity, albeit rare, include rash, itching, swelling, difficulty breathing, dizziness, nausea, and vomiting. Notably, Cerebrolysin is contraindicated in individuals allergic to pork or its products and may interact with certain medications, warranting caution in those with kidney or liver disease.

Suitable candidates for Cerebrolysin infusion encompass individuals with neurological disorders, cognitive impairment, stroke or traumatic brain injury recovery, as well as those experiencing depression or anxiety. Treatment frequency is contingent on the individual's response and condition, with daily intravenous infusions typically spanning several weeks to months.

Extensive clinical trials and studies support Cerebrolysin's efficacy, particularly in Europe and Asia where it is widely used, although it is not yet approved for use in the United States. The substance is available as a sterile intravenous solution, with recommended storage conditions involving refrigeration in a cool, dry place, shielded from light. Its preparation for intravenous infusion should be conducted by healthcare professionals according to the manufacturer's guidelines.

The half-life of Cerebrolysin is approximately 6 hours, signifying its relatively rapid metabolism and elimination from the body. When stored appropriately, Cerebrolysin maintains stability until the expiration date indicated on the packaging. This comprehensive overview underscores the intricate nature of Cerebrolysin, emphasizing its potential therapeutic value and the importance of professional guidance in its administration.

GLP-1 (A.K.A SEMAGLUTIDE)

Glucagon-like peptide-1 (GLP-1) is a naturally occurring peptide hormone secreted by intestinal L-cells in response to food intake. Its pivotal role in regulating blood sugar involves stimulating insulin secretion and reducing glucagon secretion. Additionally, GLP-1 slows gastric emptying and increases satiety, contributing to weight loss and improved glycemic control in individuals with type 2 diabetes.

The hormone is produced by intestinal L-cells, entering the bloodstream after food consumption. Its short half-life, due to rapid degradation by dipeptidyl peptidase-4 (DPP-4), necessitates the development of GLP-1 receptor agonists. These medications mimic GLP-1 effects and offer therapeutic benefits, such as enhanced glycemic control, weight loss, cardiovascular advantages, neuroprotection, and anti-inflammatory effects.

Dosage recommendations for GLP-1 receptor agonists vary, administered through injections once a day or week. These medications are employed in treating type 2 diabetes, and ongoing research explores their potential applications in obesity, cardiovascular disease, and neurodegenerative conditions. No specific signs of GLP-1 deficiency are known, as it naturally occurs in the body.

While generally well-tolerated, GLP-1 receptor agonists may cause side effects like gastrointestinal disturbances, headache, and dizziness. Contraindications include a history of pancreatitis or thyroid cancer. GLP-1 receptor agonist therapy may be suitable for individuals with uncontrolled type 2 diabetes or those at risk for cardiovascular disease.

Storage guidelines recommend refrigeration and protection from light. GLP-1 receptor agonists are injectable medications, with dosage limits varying by specific drugs and individual health statuses. Not typically administered via intravenous infusion due to its short half-life, synthetic analogs are preferred.

Treatment protocols, optimal dosages, and stability considerations depend on the specific GLP-1 receptor agonist. Semaglutide, approved for chronic weight management, exhibits higher dosages than those for diabetes treatment, proving effective in weight loss through appetite suppression and gastric effects.

Semaglutide's FDA approval in June 2021 for chronic weight management highlights its potential in obesity treatment. Clinical trials indicate promising outcomes, with participants experiencing significant weight loss. However, the medication should be part of a comprehensive weight management plan under healthcare professional supervision, considering potential side effects and risks.

Summary

Peptides have emerged as compelling candidates for potential therapeutic interventions across a spectrum of health conditions, encompassing aspects of tissue repair, growth, and cognitive and neurological function. Although the incorporation of peptides into intravenous (IV) hydration protocols for these applications is not firmly established, there is a mounting interest in exploring this avenue as a strategy to enhance the precision and efficiency of delivering these bioactive molecules. Additional research endeavors are imperative to deepen our comprehension of the safety and efficacy profiles associated with peptide-based therapies across diverse health conditions. In essence, the utilization of peptides constitutes a captivating and auspicious realm within medical research, holding the potential to introduce novel treatment modalities for a myriad of health conditions in the foreseeable future.

CHAPTER TEN
MEDICAL CONDITIONS TO ADDRESS

Disclaimer: Educational Information on Intravenous (IV) Therapy

The content provided in this section is intended solely for educational purposes. It is essential to approach this information as a foundational resource for discussion with healthcare professionals within the relevant field. The development of protocols suitable for specific clinics, clientele, and explicit approval from medical directors is imperative.

In recent years, the utilization of Intravenous (IV) therapy has gained traction, particularly among individuals exploring alternative and complementary approaches to address medical conditions. This treatment method involves administering vitamins, minerals, amino acids, and coenzymes directly into the bloodstream through intravenous infusion. IV therapy is often employed as a supplementary treatment alongside conventional medical therapies for various medical conditions.

The surge in popularity of IV therapy is attributable, in part, to its ability to facilitate the rapid delivery and absorption of essential nutrients and antioxidants. These substances may be challenging to absorb efficiently through the digestive system or may not be present in sufficient quantities in the regular diet. Individuals grappling with medical conditions that hinder nutrient absorption, such as inflammatory bowel disease, celiac disease, or those who have undergone gastric bypass surgery, can find particular benefits in IV therapy.

Moreover, individuals dealing with conditions compromising the immune system, like chronic infections or autoimmune disorders, may also derive advantages from IV therapy. This treatment modality supports cellular function, providing essential nutrients and bolstering immune system health. Chronic inflammation and pain associated with conditions like arthritis or fibromyalgia can also be alleviated through IV therapy.

The selection of vitamins, minerals, amino acids, and coenzymes in IV therapy is tailored to individual needs and the medical condition being addressed. Commonly used nutrients in IV therapy include vitamin C, magnesium, zinc, glutathione, and B-complex vitamins, chosen for their roles in supporting cellular function, reducing inflammation, and promoting overall health and wellness.

The frequency of IV therapy sessions is variable, depending on individual needs and the specific medical condition. Collaboration with healthcare professionals is strongly recommended to establish safe protocols for clients. Certain individuals may be at higher risk for adverse effects or may not be suitable candidates for IV therapy due to underlying medical conditions or medications. Nevertheless, for those who are deemed suitable candidates, IV therapy can serve as a valuable tool for supporting overall health and managing specific medical conditions.

This chapter will delve into common conditions and the associated vitamins, minerals, amino acids, and coenzymes. It is important to note that, while there is extensive research on the compounds themselves, none of the formulas for IV hydration are FDA approved for use in these patient populations. Controversy surrounds the choice between IV and oral administration of these substances, with debates centered on their effectiveness and absorption.

Oral administration is the most common method for supplementing these nutrients, but it can be limited by the digestive system's ability to absorb them, especially for individuals with compromised gut health or malabsorption issues. IV therapy, on the other hand, bypasses the digestive system, delivering nutrients directly into the bloodstream for enhanced absorption and quicker results. However, it is a more invasive, potentially more expensive, and time-consuming option compared to taking oral supplements.

Additionally, some medical professionals question the necessity of IV therapy for otherwise healthy individuals who can meet their nutritional needs through a well-balanced diet and oral supplements. Due to the lack of comprehensive research in this area, there is no conclusive argument either in favor of or against the use of IV therapy for the administration and delivery of nutrient replacements in deficiency scenarios.

Arthritis

Arthritis is a broad term encompassing more than 100 different conditions characterized by joint inflammation, affecting the joints, connective tissues, and adjacent areas. The two most prevalent forms are osteoarthritis, resulting from cartilage wear and tear, and rheumatoid arthritis, an autoimmune disorder where the body's immune system targets its own joint tissues. Manifesting as pain, stiffness, swelling, and diminished joint mobility, arthritis necessitates treatment that focuses on symptom management, improved joint function, and the prevention of further joint deterioration.

Various nutrients have been implicated in arthritis symptom management and overall joint health. Among these, vitamin D deficiency has been linked to an elevated risk of rheumatoid arthritis and osteoarthritis. Vitamin C, functioning as an antioxidant, may protect against oxidative stress and inflammation in joints. Similarly, vitamin E, another antioxidant, may aid in safeguarding joints from oxidative stress. Glucosamine and chondroitin, naturally present in cartilage, could facilitate cartilage repair and reduce inflammation in osteoarthritis patients. Omega-3 fatty acids, particularly EPA and DHA, exhibit anti-inflammatory properties, potentially mitigating inflammation in arthritis patients.

While intravenous (IV) hydration therapy is not a primary arthritis treatment, it may assist in symptom management and overall joint health. IV formulas, such as the Myers' Cocktail, comprising vitamins and minerals like vitamin C, magnesium, and B vitamins, can address nutrient deficiencies and support joint health. High-dose vitamin D infusions, administered intravenously, have been explored for their potential in reducing inflammation and supporting immune function in arthritis patients. Omega-3 fatty acid infusions, specifically EPA and DHA, may also aid in reducing inflammation.

The use of IV therapy for arthritis involves a personalized treatment protocol, considering factors like arthritis type and severity, nutritional status, and overall health. A potential schedule may include Myers' Cocktail administered once or twice a week for 4-6 weeks, followed by monthly maintenance infusions. High-dose vitamin D infusions may be administered as a single dose, followed by monthly maintenance infusions if necessary. Omega-3 fatty acid infusions may be given once or twice a month, depending on the patient's omega-3 levels and response to treatment.

Asthma

Asthma is a persistent inflammatory condition affecting the airways, characterized by recurring episodes of wheezing, breathlessness, chest tightness, and coughing. This ailment is triggered by an enhanced sensitivity of bronchial tubes to various stimuli, including allergens, irritants, infections, and exercise. These factors contribute to airway inflammation, constriction, and heightened mucus production. While asthma can affect individuals of all ages, its onset is frequently observed in childhood.

The primary objective in treating asthma is to manage inflammation and minimize symptoms, enabling patients to maintain normal activity levels and prevent acute asthma attacks. Several key nutrients have been identified as playing roles in managing asthma symptoms and promoting overall lung health. Vitamin D, for instance, has been linked to reduced asthma symptoms and improved lung function. Vitamin C, functioning as an antioxidant, may safeguard against oxidative stress and airway inflammation. Magnesium has demonstrated bronchodilatory effects, relaxing airway muscles and improving breathing. Omega-3 fatty acids possess anti-inflammatory properties, potentially reducing airway inflammation, while N-acetylcysteine (NAC), an amino acid derivative, exhibits antioxidant and mucolytic properties that may diminish mucus production and oxidative stress in asthma patients.

Although intravenous (IV) hydration therapy is not a primary treatment for asthma, it has been explored as a supportive measure for symptom management and overall lung health. Specific IV formulas have been investigated for their potential benefits in asthma patients, including the Myers' Cocktail, which combines essential vitamins and minerals, and high-dose vitamin D and NAC infusions, each tailored to address nutrient deficiencies and reduce inflammation.

The treatment protocol for asthma using IV therapy is highly individualized, taking into account factors such as symptom severity, nutritional status, and overall health. A potential treatment schedule may involve periodic administration of the Myers' Cocktail to address nutrient deficiencies and support lung health, a single high-dose vitamin D infusion, and periodic NAC infusions to reduce mucus production and oxidative stress. This approach aims to provide a comprehensive and personalized strategy for managing asthma symptoms and improving overall respiratory well-being.

Cancer

Cancer is a complex group of diseases characterized by the uncontrolled proliferation and dissemination of abnormal cells. The spectrum of cancers is extensive, encompassing various types such as breast, lung, prostate, colon, and skin cancer, among others. Although the precise etiology of cancer remains incompletely understood, a combination of genetic and environmental factors is believed to contribute to its development.

Conventional cancer treatment typically involves a multifaceted approach, incorporating surgery, radiation therapy, chemotherapy, immunotherapy, and targeted therapy. The overarching objective is to eradicate or inhibit the growth of malignant cells, prevent their metastasis, and manage associated symptoms.

Nutrition plays a pivotal role in cancer prevention, treatment, and overall health for cancer patients. Essential nutrients, including Vitamin C, known for its antioxidant properties and apoptotic effects on cancer cells, Vitamin D, which modulates cell growth and differentiation, Glutathione, a potent antioxidant combating oxidative stress, Selenium, an essential trace element with antioxidant properties, and B Vitamins (B6, B9, B12), crucial for DNA synthesis and repair, have all been implicated in these processes.

In the context of Intravenous (IV) therapy for cancer patients, while it is not a primary treatment modality, it can provide support for overall health and enhance the efficacy of conventional cancer treatments. Various IV formulas have been explored for their potential benefits, such as High-Dose Vitamin C Infusion, Glutathione IV to replenish antioxidant levels, and Vitamin and Mineral Infusion to address nutrient deficiencies and bolster overall health.

The implementation of IV therapy in cancer treatment is highly individualized and should be tailored to the unique needs of each patient. Factors influencing the treatment protocol include the type and stage of cancer, the patient's overall health status, and the specific conventional cancer treatments being administered. A potential treatment schedule may involve regular sessions of High-Dose Vitamin C Infusion and Glutathione IV, supplemented with periodic Vitamin and Mineral Infusions, all administered under the supervision of a healthcare professional with expertise in cancer care.

Chronic Fatigue Syndrome

Chronic Fatigue Syndrome (CFS), alternatively known as Myalgic Encephalomyelitis (ME), is a multifaceted and incapacitating disorder characterized by persistent, unexplained fatigue that remains unaffected by rest and may exacerbate with physical or mental activity. Although the precise etiology of CFS remains incompletely understood, it is postulated to result from a confluence of genetic, environmental, and immune factors. Manifestations of this syndrome encompass muscle pain, joint pain, sleep disturbances, cognitive impairments, and post-exertional malaise. The therapeutic approach to CFS typically revolves around symptom management and enhancement of overall quality of life.

Numerous nutrients have been implicated in the management of chronic fatigue, including Vitamin B12, which has been correlated with fatigue and cognitive challenges. Supplementation of Vitamin B12 may ameliorate energy levels and cognitive function in certain CFS patients. Vitamin C, functioning as an antioxidant, safeguards cells from oxidative stress and may enhance overall immune function in individuals with CFS. Coenzyme Q10, playing a pivotal role in cellular energy production, could potentially alleviate fatigue in CFS patients. Magnesium, essential for energy production and muscle function, is associated with fatigue and muscle pain in some CFS patients when present in low levels. L-Carnitine, an amino acid derivative facilitating the transport of fatty acids into mitochondria for energy production, might contribute to fatigue reduction in CFS patients.

While there is no cure for CFS, intravenous (IV) hydration therapy emerges as a potential means of symptom management and overall health support. Various IV formulas have been explored for CFS, including the Myers' Cocktail, a blend of vitamins and minerals addressing nutrient deficiencies and promoting overall health. Additionally, high-dose Vitamin B12 infusions administered intravenously may improve energy levels and cognitive function. The combination of CoQ10 and L-Carnitine in infusion form could potentially support energy production and reduce fatigue in CFS patients.

The application of IV therapy in the treatment protocol for CFS is highly personalized, contingent upon individual patient needs encompassing symptom severity, nutritional status, and overall health. A conceivable treatment schedule might involve regular Myers' Cocktail infusions, Vitamin B12 infusions based on the patient's B12 levels and response to treatment, and a course of CoQ10 and L-Carnitine infusions to support energy production and alleviate fatigue. This structured approach aims to provide a comprehensive and tailored therapeutic strategy for individuals grappling with the challenges of Chronic Fatigue Syndrome.

Chronic Pain

Chronic pain is characterized by persistent or recurrent discomfort lasting beyond the typical healing period, typically enduring for more than three months. Its etiology can be multifaceted, stemming from factors such as injury, infection, inflammation, nerve damage, or an underlying medical condition. The scope of chronic pain is extensive, impacting any part of the body and manifesting as either constant or intermittent. Its severity ranges from mild to severe, significantly influencing an individual's quality of life by contributing to sleep disturbances, depression, and reduced physical functioning.

In the context of chronic pain management, various nutrients, including vitamins, minerals, amino acids, and coenzymes, play pivotal roles in symptom alleviation and overall pain regulation. For instance, vitamin D deficiency has been correlated with heightened pain sensitivity and chronic pain conditions, such as fibromyalgia and chronic low back pain. Supplementation with vitamin D may mitigate inflammation, bolster immune function, and modulate pain perception.

Magnesium, essential for nerve function and muscle relaxation, is implicated in chronic pain conditions like fibromyalgia and migraines. Supplementation with magnesium may help alleviate pain and muscle tension. B vitamins, specifically thiamine, pyridoxine, and cobalamin, contribute to nerve function and neurotransmitter synthesis involved in pain regulation. Supplementation with B vitamins may reduce neuropathic pain and enhance nerve function. Alpha-lipoic acid (ALA), an antioxidant, may protect against oxidative stress and inflammation, showing promise in treating neuropathic pain, particularly in diabetic neuropathy patients.

While intravenous (IV) hydration therapy is not a primary treatment for chronic pain, it can assist in symptom management and overall pain regulation. Notable IV formulas include the Myers' Cocktail, a blend of vitamins and minerals, the High-Dose Vitamin D Infusion for its potential anti-inflammatory properties, and Magnesium Infusion to alleviate pain and muscle tension.

IV therapy for chronic pain involves a highly individualized treatment protocol tailored to each patient's specific needs, considering factors such as symptom severity, nutritional status, and overall health. A potential treatment schedule might include Myers' Cocktail administered once or twice a week for 4-6 weeks, followed by monthly maintenance infusions. High-Dose Vitamin D Infusion could be administered as a single high-dose infusion, with monthly maintenance infusions if necessary. Magnesium Infusion might be administered once or twice a month based on the patient's magnesium levels and response to treatment, specifically targeting pain and muscle tension relief.

Concussions

A concussion, categorized as a mild traumatic brain injury (TBI), occurs due to a sudden impact or jolt to the head or body, resulting in the rapid movement of the brain within the skull. This movement can trigger chemical changes in the brain, potentially causing the stretching or damage of brain cells. The manifestation of concussions encompasses a spectrum of symptoms, including headache, confusion, dizziness, nausea, and momentary loss of consciousness. Recovery periods vary, with most individuals fully recuperating within days to weeks. However, repeated concussions may lead to lasting effects on cognitive function and an increased susceptibility to chronic traumatic encephalopathy (CTE).

Numerous nutrients have been implicated in the recovery and management of concussions. Among these, Omega-3 Fatty Acids play a critical role in reducing inflammation and facilitating brain cell repair. Vitamin D exhibits neuroprotective effects and may aid in the post-concussion recovery process. Magnesium, essential for proper nerve and muscle function, may help mitigate the risk of post-concussion symptoms. Vitamin C, an antioxidant, safeguards the brain from oxidative stress and bolsters the immune system. B Vitamins, including B6, B9, and B12, are crucial for maintaining optimal brain function and promoting recovery.

In the absence of a specific treatment for concussions, Intravenous (IV) hydration therapy has been explored to support overall health and recovery. Notable IV formulas for concussion management include the Myers' Cocktail, a blend of vitamins and minerals that may address nutrient deficiencies and enhance overall health. High-dose vitamin D infusion, aimed at supporting neuroprotection and recovery post-concussion, is administered within the first week, with potential monthly maintenance infusions. Omega-3 Fatty Acid Infusion, administered weekly for 2-4 weeks, is intended to support brain cell repair and alleviate inflammation.

The treatment protocol using IV therapy is highly individualized, tailored to the specific needs of each patient. Considerations include the severity of symptoms, nutritional status, and overall health. A potential treatment schedule involves the administration of the Myers' Cocktail within the first 24-72 hours after the concussion, followed by once or twice a week for 2-4 weeks. Vitamin D infusion, given as a single high-dose within the first week, may be followed by monthly maintenance infusions if necessary. Omega-3 Fatty Acid Infusion, administered once a week for 2-4 weeks, aims to support brain cell repair and reduce inflammation.

It is crucial to note that a high-dose vitamin D infusion involves a substantial amount of vitamin D delivered intravenously, with potential risks including hypercalcemia, kidney stones, and gastrointestinal symptoms. Individuals with specific medical conditions, such as hyperparathyroidism or kidney disease, should exercise caution. Omega-3 infusion, delivering high doses of essential fatty acids, should only be administered under the supervision of a qualified healthcare professional. Potential side effects include allergic reactions, gastrointestinal upset, and bleeding disorders. Patients considering omega-3 infusion should discuss potential risks and benefits with their healthcare provider, emphasizing the need for further research to fully understand its safety and effectiveness across various medical conditions.

Chronic Obstructive Pulmonary Disease (COPD)

Chronic Obstructive Pulmonary Disease (COPD) is a collective term encompassing a group of progressive lung conditions, such as emphysema and chronic bronchitis, which manifest as airflow obstruction and respiratory challenges. The predominant cause of COPD is prolonged exposure to irritating gases or particulate matter, with cigarette smoke standing out as the most prevalent offender. The condition is characterized by persistent inflammation, airway remodeling, and oxidative stress, culminating in diminished lung function and breathlessness. The therapeutic approach to COPD centers on symptom management, enhancement of lung function, and the prevention of exacerbations.

Various nutrients have been implicated in the management of COPD symptoms and overall pulmonary well-being. Among these, Vitamin D plays a crucial role, as low levels have been linked to decreased lung function and heightened risk of exacerbations in COPD patients. Supplementation of Vitamin D may mitigate inflammation, fortify immune function, and enhance overall lung health. Additionally, Vitamin C, functioning as an antioxidant, may safeguard against oxidative stress and inflammation in the airways, potentially ameliorating COPD symptoms. Vitamin E, another antioxidant, is posited to protect against oxidative stress and inflammation in the airways, potentially alleviating COPD symptoms. N-acetylcysteine (NAC), an amino acid derivative and glutathione precursor, possesses antioxidant and mucolytic properties that may alleviate mucus production and oxidative stress in COPD patients. Magnesium has been observed to exhibit bronchodilatory effects, potentially relaxing airway muscles and ameliorating breathing difficulties in COPD patients.

While intravenous (IV) hydration therapy is not a primary treatment modality for COPD, it may contribute to symptom management and overall pulmonary health support. Noteworthy IV formulas explored for

COPD patients include the Myers' Cocktail, a blend of vitamins and minerals designed to address nutrient deficiencies and support overall lung health. High-dose Vitamin D infusion administered intravenously has been investigated for its potential in reducing inflammation and supporting immune function in COPD patients. N-acetylcysteine (NAC) infusion through IV administration may assist in reducing mucus production and oxidative stress in COPD patients.

The implementation of an IV therapy protocol for COPD treatment is highly individualized and should be tailored to the specific needs of each patient. Factors such as the severity of symptoms, nutritional status, and overall health must be taken into account. A proposed treatment schedule could involve periodic Myers' Cocktail infusions, administered once or twice a week for 4-6 weeks, followed by monthly maintenance infusions to sustain overall lung health and address nutrient deficiencies. High-dose Vitamin D infusion may be considered as a single high-dose administration, followed by monthly maintenance infusions if necessary, contingent on the patient's vitamin D levels and response to treatment. N-acetylcysteine (NAC) infusion could be administered once or twice a month to diminish mucus production and oxidative stress, thereby contributing to the management of COPD symptoms.

Fibromyalgia

Fibromyalgia, a persistent pain disorder, is characterized by widespread musculoskeletal pain, fatigue, sleep disturbances, and cognitive challenges. Although the exact etiology remains incompletely understood, it is widely believed to be influenced by a combination of genetic, environmental, and immune factors. Fibromyalgia is thought to emanate from aberrant pain processing within the central nervous system, resulting in an elevated sensitivity to pain. The primary focus of fibromyalgia treatment typically revolves around symptom management and enhancing overall quality of life.

Various nutrients have been implicated in alleviating fibromyalgia symptoms. Among these, Vitamin D is associated with lower fibromyalgia levels, and supplementation may alleviate pain and enhance overall health. Magnesium deficiency is linked to symptoms such as muscle pain, fatigue, and sleep disturbances in fibromyalgia patients, and supplementation may ameliorate these manifestations. Vitamin B12 deficiency is also associated with fatigue and cognitive difficulties common in fibromyalgia, and supplementation may improve energy levels and cognitive function. Coenzyme Q10, which plays a role in cellular energy production and possesses antioxidant properties, is observed at low levels in fibromyalgia patients, and supplementation may reduce fatigue and pain. L-carnitine, an amino acid derivative involved in energy production, may also help alleviate fatigue and pain in fibromyalgia patients.

While there is no cure for fibromyalgia, intravenous (IV) hydration therapy may assist in managing symptoms and supporting overall health. Some investigated IV formulas for fibromyalgia include the Myers' Cocktail, a blend of vitamins and minerals; magnesium infusion, shown to reduce pain and improve sleep; and a vitamin and mineral infusion, combining essential nutrients to address deficiencies.

The treatment protocol for fibromyalgia using IV therapy is highly individualized, considering factors such as symptom severity, nutritional status, and overall health. A potential treatment schedule may involve Myers' Cocktail administered once or twice a week for 4-6 weeks, followed by monthly maintenance infusions. Magnesium infusion may include a single high-dose infusion, followed by monthly maintenance infusions if necessary. Vitamin and mineral infusion may be administered once or twice a month to address nutrient deficiencies and support overall health.

Immunological Disorders

Immunological disorders encompass a spectrum of conditions characterized by the malfunctioning of the immune system. These disorders are broadly categorized into three main classes: immunodeficiencies, autoimmune diseases, and hypersensitivity reactions. Immunodeficiencies manifest when the immune system is incapable of mounting an effective defense against infections and diseases. Autoimmune diseases, on the other hand, entail the immune system mistakenly attacking the body's own tissues, misconstruing them as foreign invaders. Hypersensitivity reactions, exemplified by allergies, occur when the immune system excessively responds to otherwise innocuous substances.

The treatment modalities for immunological disorders are diverse and contingent upon the specific condition. Interventions may include medications, immunotherapy, or lifestyle adjustments aimed at symptom management and overall enhancement of immune function.

Nutrients such as vitamins, minerals, amino acids, and coenzymes play pivotal roles in supporting immune function and may contribute to the development or treatment of immunological disorders. Vitamin C, a robust antioxidant, is essential for various cellular functions and collagen synthesis, crucial for tissue and organ integrity. Vitamin D regulates immune function, and deficiencies have been linked to various immunological disorders. Zinc, an essential trace element, participates in immune functions such as cell division, gene expression, and inflammation regulation. Deficiency in zinc has been associated with compromised immune responses. Glutathione, a potent antioxidant, helps maintain cellular oxidation-reduction balance critical for proper immune function.

While intravenous (IV) hydration therapy is not a primary treatment for immunological disorders, it can address nutrient deficiencies and support overall immune function. Customized nutrient infusions, incorporating vitamins C and D, zinc, and glutathione, aim to address individual nutrient deficiencies. The Myer's Cocktail, a well-known IV formula, combines B vitamins, vitamin C, magnesium, and calcium, potentially enhancing immune function and mitigating inflammation.

The IV therapy protocol for immunological disorders is highly individualized, considering factors such as the disorder type and severity, nutritional status, and overall health. A potential treatment schedule may involve customized nutrient infusions or Myer's Cocktail administered once or twice a month, tailored based on regular monitoring of nutrient levels and symptom management. Adjustments to the treatment schedule can be made based on the patient's response to the therapy.

Infertility

Infertility is a complex medical condition characterized by the inability to conceive a child following one year of consistent, unprotected sexual intercourse. This condition can impact both men and women and may arise from various factors, encompassing hormonal imbalances, structural abnormalities, genetic disorders, and environmental influences. Infertility can originate from issues within the female reproductive system, the male reproductive system, or a combination of both, and in some instances, the root cause remains unidentified.

Several key nutrients, including vitamins, minerals, amino acids, and coenzymes, play pivotal roles in supporting fertility by contributing to reproductive health, hormonal equilibrium, and overall well-being. For instance, folic acid, an essential B vitamin, is crucial for DNA synthesis and cell division, playing a vital role in the development of a healthy embryo. Vitamin D, essential for hormone production and regulation, has been linked to infertility in both men and women when deficient.

Coenzyme Q10 (CoQ10), an antioxidant, aids in cellular energy production and may enhance sperm quality and female reproductive health. Omega-3 fatty acids, possessing anti-inflammatory properties, can potentially support hormonal balance and overall reproductive health.

While intravenous (IV) hydration therapy is not a primary treatment for infertility, it can address nutrient deficiencies and contribute to overall health in individuals attempting to conceive. Various IV formulas have been explored for infertility, such as a customized nutrient infusion that includes folic acid, vitamin D, CoQ10, and omega-3 fatty acids. The Myer's Cocktail, a well-known IV formula comprising B vitamins, vitamin C, magnesium, and calcium, may also be utilized to enhance overall health and support fertility.

The treatment protocol involving IV therapy for infertility is highly personalized, taking into account factors such as the severity of infertility, nutritional status, and overall health. A potential treatment schedule may involve periodic administration of customized nutrient infusions or Myer's Cocktail, tailored to the patient's specific nutrient deficiencies and response to treatment. This schedule can be adjusted based on regular monitoring of nutrient levels and overall reproductive health.

Inflammatory Bowel Disorders

Inflammatory bowel disorders (IBD) encompass a spectrum of chronic inflammatory conditions that impact the gastrointestinal tract. The prevalent forms of IBD include Crohn's disease, which can affect any part of the gastrointestinal tract, and ulcerative colitis, which specifically targets the colon and rectum. Both conditions entail an aberrant immune response, resulting in inflammation and damage to the lining of the intestines. Manifestations of IBD encompass abdominal pain, diarrhea, fatigue, weight loss, and malnutrition. The comprehensive management of IBD typically entails a combination of medications to mitigate inflammation, surgical interventions, and lifestyle adjustments aimed at minimizing symptoms.

Patients grappling with IBD often encounter nutrient deficiencies due to factors such as malabsorption, inflammation, or dietary restrictions. Essential nutrients play a pivotal role in managing IBD symptoms and promoting overall health. Notable among these nutrients are:

1. **Vitamin D**: This vitamin is integral to immune function and may exhibit anti-inflammatory properties. Many individuals with IBD exhibit low levels of vitamin D, which can predispose them to bone loss and heightened susceptibility to infections.

2. **Vitamin B12**: Essential for red blood cell production and neurological function, vitamin B12 is frequently malabsorbed in individuals with Crohn's disease, particularly those who have undergone ileal resections.

3. **Iron**: Crucial for red blood cell production and oxygen transport, iron deficiency anemia is commonplace in IBD patients owing to blood loss and malabsorption linked to inflammation.

4. **Zinc**: Involved in immune function, wound healing, and tissue repair, zinc deficiencies may arise in individuals with IBD due to malabsorption, increased intestinal loss, or reduced intake.

5. **Glutamine**: This amino acid serves as an energy source for intestinal cells and may aid in maintaining the integrity of the intestinal barrier.

To address nutrient deficiencies and dehydration in IBD patients, intravenous (IV) hydration therapy has been explored. Various IV formulas have been proposed, including customized nutrient infusions and glutamine infusions, which aim to tailor the treatment to individual nutrient deficiencies and support overall health.

The treatment protocol utilizing IV therapy for IBD is highly personalized, taking into account factors such as the type and severity of IBD, nutritional status, and overall health. A potential treatment schedule may involve customized nutrient infusions administered once or twice a month, with adjustments based on regular monitoring of nutrient levels and symptom management. Glutamine infusions may be administered once or twice a week for 4-6 weeks, followed by a maintenance schedule contingent upon the patient's response to treatment and overall health. This approach seeks to optimize therapeutic outcomes and enhance the quality of life for individuals navigating the challenges of IBD.

Lupus

Lupus is a chronic autoimmune disorder characterized by the immune system's misguided attack on healthy tissues, resulting in inflammation and damage to various organs and systems within the body, including the skin, joints, kidneys, heart, lungs, and blood vessels. Systemic lupus erythematosus (SLE) stands out as the most prevalent form among various types of lupus. The precise etiology of lupus remains incompletely understood, yet it is widely acknowledged to involve a complex interplay of genetic, environmental, and hormonal factors.

The management of lupus predominantly centers on symptom control, inflammation reduction, and prevention of organ damage. In the realm of nutritional considerations for lupus patients, various vitamins, minerals, amino acids, and coenzymes have been implicated in symptom alleviation and overall health improvement. Vitamin D, for instance, has been associated with lupus, and supplementation may contribute to inflammation reduction, immune function support, and enhanced overall health in select patients. Omega-3 fatty acids, recognized for their anti-inflammatory properties, may similarly aid in mitigating inflammation and enhancing cardiovascular health in individuals with lupus.

Antioxidants, including vitamin C, vitamin E, and glutathione, have demonstrated potential in shielding cells from oxidative stress, a factor believed to contribute to inflammation and organ damage in lupus patients. B vitamins, such as B6, B9 (folate), and B12, play pivotal roles in immune function and may contribute to overall health improvement in lupus patients. Additionally, selenium, an essential trace element with antioxidant properties, is believed to offer protection against oxidative stress in individuals with lupus.

While intravenous (IV) hydration therapy does not serve as the primary treatment for lupus, it may play a supportive role in symptom management and overall health maintenance. Specific IV formulas explored for lupus patients encompass the Myers' Cocktail, a blend of vitamins and minerals designed to address nutrient deficiencies and support overall health. High-dose vitamin D infusion administered intravenously has been investigated for its potential to reduce inflammation and bolster immune function in lupus patients. Another explored option is an antioxidant infusion, combining vitamin C, vitamin E, and glutathione to protect against oxidative stress and promote overall health in individuals with lupus.

The utilization of IV therapy in lupus treatment adheres to a highly individualized approach, tailoring the protocol to each patient's unique needs. Considerations include the severity of symptoms, nutritional status, and overall health. A prospective treatment schedule may involve Myers' Cocktail administered once or twice a week for 4-6 weeks, followed by monthly maintenance infusions for ongoing health support and nutrient replenishment. High-dose vitamin D infusion could be administered as a single high-dose infusion, followed by periodic maintenance infusions based on the patient's vitamin D levels and response to treatment. Antioxidant infusions may be recommended once or twice a month to fortify against oxidative stress and maintain overall health in lupus patients.

Menstruation

Menstruation, a natural physiological process occurring in females of reproductive age, is characterized by the cyclic shedding of the uterine lining (endometrium) in response to hormonal fluctuations when pregnancy does not transpire. Typically commencing during adolescence and persisting until menopause, the menstrual cycle spans around 28 days, yet considerable variations exist among individuals. Alongside this biological phenomenon come an array of physical and emotional symptoms, including but not limited to cramps, bloating, fatigue, and mood swings. While menstruation is considered a normal aspect of a woman's life, some may encounter severe symptoms necessitating medical intervention or supportive care.

Several essential nutrients, namely Iron, Vitamin B6, Magnesium, and Calcium, play pivotal roles in supporting overall health during menstruation and may contribute to the alleviation of associated symptoms. Iron, for instance, is crucial for replenishing blood lost during menstruation, reducing the risk of anemia and maintaining healthy red blood cells. Vitamin B6 is involved in neurotransmitter production, potentially mitigating mood swings and emotional symptoms. Magnesium, vital for muscle and nerve function, may help alleviate menstrual cramps, while Calcium contributes to bone health and may alleviate premenstrual symptoms such as mood swings, bloating, and cramping.

In the realm of medical interventions, while intravenous (IV) hydration therapy is not a primary treatment for menstruation, it can address nutrient deficiencies and support overall health during the menstrual cycle. Customized nutrient infusions and the well-known Myer's Cocktail, both containing a blend of essential vitamins, minerals, and amino acids, have been explored for their potential in improving overall health and alleviating menstrual symptoms.

The treatment protocol for menstruation utilizing IV therapy is highly individualized, contingent upon factors such as the severity of menstrual symptoms, nutritional status, and overall health. A potential treatment schedule might involve administering a customized nutrient infusion or Myer's Cocktail once or twice a month, contingent upon the patient's specific nutrient deficiencies and response to treatment. Regular monitoring of nutrient levels and symptom management would inform any necessary adjustments to the treatment schedule.

Migraines

A migraine is a complex neurological condition characterized by moderate to severe headaches, frequently accompanied by symptoms such as nausea, vomiting, and heightened sensitivity to light and sound. These debilitating migraine attacks can persist for varying durations, ranging from a few hours to several days. The exact etiology of migraines remains incompletely understood, but a combination of genetic and environmental factors is believed to contribute to their onset. The pathophysiological mechanisms underlying migraines involve intricate changes in brain chemistry, inflammation, and the dilation and constriction of blood vessels within the brain.

Various essential nutrients, including magnesium, vitamin B2 (Riboflavin), coenzyme Q10, and vitamin D, have been implicated in the prevention and management of migraines. Magnesium deficiency, for instance, has been associated with migraines, and supplementing with magnesium may serve to prevent or diminish the frequency and severity of migraine attacks. Riboflavin, essential for brain energy production, has demonstrated efficacy in reducing the frequency and severity of migraines in certain individuals. Coenzyme Q10, with its involvement in brain energy production and antioxidant properties, has shown promise in reducing migraine frequency. Additionally, vitamin D, with its anti-inflammatory properties, may modulate pain pathways in the brain and potentially mitigate migraines.

In the realm of migraine management, intravenous (IV) hydration therapy has emerged as a supportive measure to alleviate symptoms and promote overall health. Notably, specific IV formulas have been explored for their potential efficacy in migraine treatment. The Myers' Cocktail, a blend of vitamins and minerals, including magnesium, B vitamins, and vitamin C, addresses nutrient deficiencies and supports overall health, providing relief during acute migraine episodes. High-dose magnesium infusion administered intravenously has demonstrated effectiveness in reducing the severity and duration of acute migraine attacks. Furthermore, a vitamin and mineral infusion, incorporating essential nutrients such as vitamin D, riboflavin, and CoQ10, may contribute to overall health and address nutrient deficiencies in individuals affected by migraines.

The implementation of IV therapy for migraines involves a highly personalized treatment protocol tailored to the unique needs of each patient. Factors considered in this individualized approach include the severity of symptoms, nutritional status, and overall health. A potential treatment schedule may include the administration of the Myers' Cocktail during acute migraine attacks to provide relief and support overall health. High-dose magnesium infusions may be administered during acute episodes or as a preventive measure at regular intervals, depending on the patient's magnesium levels and response to treatment. Additionally, vitamin and mineral infusions may be recommended once or twice a month to address nutrient deficiencies and promote overall health in individuals affected by migraines.

Mood Disorders

Mood disorders, also recognized as affective disorders, represent a category of mental health conditions characterized by disruptions in mood, spanning from profound depression to heightened mania. Prevalent mood disorders encompass major depressive disorder (MDD), bipolar disorder, and persistent depressive disorder (dysthymia). While the precise etiology of mood disorders remains incompletely understood, a multifaceted interplay of genetic, biological, environmental, and psychological factors is perceived to contribute to their manifestation. Treatment for mood disorders typically integrates a multifaceted approach involving medication, psychotherapy, and lifestyle adjustments, all aimed at symptom management and enhancement of overall well-being.

Within the realm of mood disorders, emerging evidence suggests the involvement of specific nutrients in their development, progression, and therapeutic intervention. Notably, deficiencies in Vitamin D have been correlated with depression and mood disorders, given its integral role in various brain processes, including neurotransmitter synthesis crucial for mood regulation. B vitamins, particularly B6, B9 (folate), and B12, are deemed essential for proper brain function and neurotransmitter synthesis, with deficiencies linked to mood disorders such as depression. Magnesium, vital for numerous biochemical processes, including mood regulation, has shown associations with depression and anxiety when its levels are low. Amino acids like tryptophan and tyrosine, acting as precursors to neurotransmitters such as serotonin, dopamine, and norepinephrine, play pivotal roles in mood regulation.

While intravenous (IV) hydration therapy is not a primary modality for treating mood disorders, it can be instrumental in addressing nutrient deficiencies and supporting overall mental health. Customized nutrient infusions, encompassing a tailored blend of vitamins, minerals, and amino acids, as well as well-established IV formulas like the Myer's Cocktail,

have been explored for their potential efficacy in improving mood and
energy levels in certain individuals.

The implementation of IV therapy for mood disorders adheres to a highly
individualized treatment protocol, contingent upon factors such as the
specific type and severity of the mood disorder, the patient's nutritional
status, and overall health. A conceivable treatment schedule may involve
periodic administration of customized nutrient infusions or Myer's
Cocktail, with the frequency adjusted based on ongoing monitoring of
nutrient levels and the patient's response to treatment. This approach
underscores the personalized nature of IV therapy in the context of mood
disorder management.

Parkinson's Disease

It is a progressive neurological disorder, significantly impacts the motor system, resulting in challenges related to movement, muscle stiffness, and compromised balance. This condition is primarily characterized by the gradual loss of dopamine-producing neurons in the substantia nigra, a critical brain region responsible for coordinating movement. While the precise cause of neuronal degeneration in Parkinson's Disease remains incompletely understood, there is consensus that both genetic and environmental factors contribute to its development.

Common symptoms associated with Parkinson's Disease encompass tremors, bradykinesia (slowed movement), rigidity, and postural instability. The exploration of vitamins, minerals, amino acids, and coenzymes in the context of Parkinson's Disease reveals their potential implications in both its pathogenesis and treatment.

Vitamin B6, or Pyridoxine, plays a vital role in dopamine and neurotransmitter synthesis, with low levels linked to an elevated risk of Parkinson's Disease. Vitamin E, a potent antioxidant, is instrumental in shielding cells from oxidative stress, believed to contribute to dopaminergic neuron degeneration. Coenzyme Q10, a key component in the mitochondrial electron transport chain, exhibits reduced levels in the mitochondria of Parkinson's patients, impacting cellular energy production. Glutathione, a powerful antioxidant composed of glutamate, cysteine, and glycine, experiences decreased levels in the substantia nigra of individuals with Parkinson's Disease. Additionally, recent studies suggest a correlation between low levels of Vitamin D and an increased risk of developing Parkinson's Disease, with Vitamin D exerting neuroprotective effects and modulating immune responses in the brain.

In the realm of therapeutic interventions, while there is no cure for Parkinson's Disease, Intravenous (IV) hydration therapy emerges as a potential avenue for symptom management and overall health support. Various IV formulas have been explored for their potential benefits in Parkinson's Disease management.

High-dose glutathione delivered intravenously is proposed to replenish brain glutathione levels and mitigate oxidative stress. A Vitamin and Mineral Infusion, incorporating essential nutrients such as Vitamins B6, E, and D, as well as minerals like magnesium and zinc, aims to address nutrient deficiencies and promote overall health in Parkinson's patients. Amino Acid Infusion, including L-tyrosine as a dopamine precursor and L-carnitine supporting mitochondrial function, may be included to bolster neurotransmitter production and cellular energy metabolism.

The application of IV therapy for Parkinson's Disease follows a highly individualized treatment protocol, taking into account factors such as symptom severity, nutritional status, and overall health. The suggested treatment schedule involves periodic sessions of Glutathione IV, Vitamin and Mineral Infusion, and Amino Acid Infusion based on the patient's specific needs and response to treatment. This tailored approach underscores the nuanced nature of addressing Parkinson's Disease through IV therapy interventions.

Polycystic ovary syndrome (PCOS)

Polycystic ovary syndrome (PCOS) stands as a prevalent hormonal disorder that affects women in their reproductive years. The condition is characterized by an intricate imbalance of reproductive hormones, resulting in the formation of small cysts in the ovaries, irregular menstrual periods, and elevated levels of androgens, commonly known as male hormones. This hormonal disarray manifests in various symptomatic expressions, including but not limited to infertility, hirsutism (excessive hair growth), acne, weight gain, and insulin resistance. PCOS is a multifaceted health issue influenced by a combination of genetic predisposition and lifestyle choices.

Within the realm of PCOS management, certain nutrients have been identified to play crucial roles in supporting overall health and mitigating specific symptoms or complications associated with the condition. Inositol, a vitamin-like substance, has exhibited efficacy in enhancing insulin sensitivity, regulating hormone levels, and improving ovarian function in women with PCOS. Vitamin D deficiency, commonly observed in PCOS cases, may contribute to insulin resistance and hormonal imbalances. Chromium, an essential trace element, proves valuable in enhancing insulin sensitivity and glucose metabolism among PCOS patients. Additionally, magnesium, a participant in various physiological processes, including glucose metabolism, has shown promise in ameliorating insulin resistance in women with PCOS.

While intravenous (IV) hydration therapy is not a primary treatment for PCOS, it can serve as a supportive measure by addressing nutrient deficiencies and promoting overall health in affected women. Notable IV formulas investigated for PCOS include the Customized Nutrient Infusion, tailored to address individual nutrient deficiencies with a blend of vitamins, minerals, and amino acids, and the Myer's Cocktail, a well-known formula featuring a combination of B vitamins, vitamin C, magnesium, and calcium, which may contribute to improved overall health and relief from certain PCOS symptoms.

The application of IV therapy in the treatment protocol for PCOS is highly individualized, necessitating customization based on factors such as the severity of symptoms, nutritional status, and overall health of each patient. A potential treatment schedule involves administering the Customized Nutrient Infusion or Myer's Cocktail once or twice a month, with adjustments based on regular monitoring of nutrient levels and symptom management. This tailored approach ensures a comprehensive and effective strategy for managing PCOS through IV therapy.

Postoperative Period

The post-surgical or postoperative period, denoting the interval subsequent to a surgical intervention, is a pivotal phase in the patient's recuperative journey. This period assumes paramount significance as it involves vigilant monitoring of vital signs, meticulous pain management, complication prevention, and facilitation of the healing process. The temporal extent of the post-surgical period is contingent upon diverse factors, including the nature of the surgery, the patient's overall health condition, and the potential emergence of complications.

An integral aspect of post-surgical recovery lies in the recognition of the pivotal role played by specific nutrients, namely Vitamins, Minerals, Amino Acids, and Coenzymes, in fostering healing, bolstering immune function, and ensuring overall well-being. Vitamin C, for instance, is indispensable for collagen synthesis, tissue repair, and immune fortification. Vitamin A supports epithelial cell growth, wound healing, and immune function. B Vitamins are crucial for energy production, immune function, and tissue repair. Zinc contributes to protein synthesis, cell division, and wound healing. Glutamine, an amino acid implicated in immune function and intestinal health, may experience depletion during surgery and stress. Arginine, another amino acid, aids in wound healing and immune support.

In the realm of post-operative care, Intravenous (IV) hydration therapy emerges as a valuable adjunct by delivering essential nutrients critical for recovery and fortifying immune function. Prominent among these IV formulas are the Myer's Cocktail, a blend of B vitamins, vitamin C, magnesium, and calcium known for its potential to support overall health and recovery. Additionally, the Immune Boost Infusion offers a customized array of nutrients, including vitamin C, vitamin A, zinc, glutamine, and arginine, specifically designed to fortify immune function and promote wound healing.

Developing a coherent treatment protocol utilizing IV therapy in post-surgical patients necessitates a personalized approach, accounting for factors such as the specific type of surgery, the patient's overall health status, and nutritional profile. A plausible treatment schedule may encompass the administration of either the Myer's Cocktail or Immune Boost Infusion within the initial 24-48 hours post-surgery, with subsequent infusions tailored to the patient's recovery trajectory and response to treatment. This individualized approach ensures optimal support for post-surgical recovery, emphasizing the significance of tailored nutritional interventions in augmenting the healing process.

Preoperative Period

The pre-surgical period, commonly referred to as the preoperative period, constitutes the timeframe preceding a surgical intervention. This phase involves a comprehensive assessment of patients, encompassing their overall health, medical history, and potential risks associated with the impending surgery. It holds paramount importance in optimizing patient health to ensure the best possible condition for the surgery, thereby contributing to enhanced surgical outcomes and a reduction in complications.

Within the realm of pre-surgical preparation, certain essential nutrients, including vitamins, minerals, amino acids, and coenzymes, play a pivotal role in priming the body for the impending surgical procedure. Vitamin C, vital for collagen synthesis, tissue repair, and immune function, stands as a crucial component. Additionally, Vitamin A supports epithelial cell growth, wound healing, and immune function. B Vitamins are integral for energy production, immune function, and tissue repair, while zinc plays a significant role in protein synthesis, cell division, and wound healing. Glutamine, an amino acid involved in immune function and intestinal health, and arginine, supporting wound healing and immune function, are also noteworthy in this context.

In the realm of pre-surgical care, intravenous (IV) hydration therapy emerges as a valuable intervention. By delivering essential nutrients directly into the bloodstream, IV therapy aims to optimize patient health and fortify immune function. Notable IV formulas employed in pre-surgical patients include the Myer's Cocktail, a blend of B vitamins, vitamin C, magnesium, and calcium, promoting overall health and recovery. Another formulation, the Immune Boost Infusion, is customized to include nutrients specifically supporting immune function and wound healing, such as vitamin C, vitamin A, zinc, glutamine, and arginine.

The implementation of IV therapy in pre-surgical patients necessitates a personalized treatment protocol tailored to individual needs. This protocol may vary based on factors such as the type of surgery, the patient's overall health, and nutritional status. A suggested treatment schedule could involve administering the Myer's Cocktail or Immune Boost Infusion 1-2 weeks before surgery, with additional infusions administered as needed, guided by the patient's response to treatment and recommendations from the surgical team. This meticulous approach to pre-surgical care underscores the commitment to optimizing patient health and fostering positive surgical outcomes.

Ulcers

Ulcers are characterized as open sores that can manifest on either the skin or mucous membranes. Among the various types of ulcers, the most prevalent is the peptic ulcer, which emerges in the lining of the stomach, esophagus, or upper section of the small intestine. The development of peptic ulcers is typically attributed to an imbalance between the stomach's acid production and its inherent defensive mechanisms. This imbalance often arises from factors such as infection with the bacterium Helicobacter pylori (H. pylori) or the utilization of nonsteroidal anti-inflammatory drugs (NSAIDs). Common symptoms associated with ulcers encompass abdominal pain, bloating, nausea, and weight loss.

The conventional approach to ulcer treatment involves a combination of medications to diminish stomach acid, antibiotics to combat H. pylori infections, and lifestyle adjustments to facilitate healing and prevent recurrence. Furthermore, various nutrients play pivotal roles in the healing process of ulcers and the overall health of the gastrointestinal system. These include antioxidants such as Vitamin C, essential for collagen production and potentially eradicating H. pylori infections. Zinc, contributing to immune function and tissue repair, may aid ulcer healing and maintain gastrointestinal lining integrity. Glutamine, an amino acid, serves as an energy source for intestinal cells and may contribute to the preservation of gastrointestinal lining integrity. Vitamin A is crucial for maintaining the mucosal lining of the gastrointestinal tract, offering support for ulcer healing.

Although intravenous (IV) hydration therapy is not the primary treatment for ulcers, it can effectively address nutrient deficiencies and support overall gastrointestinal health. Specific IV formulas designed for ulcer management include customized nutrient infusions, blending vitamins and minerals to address individual deficiencies and support gastrointestinal health. Additionally, glutamine infusions administered intravenously may promote intestinal barrier function and contribute to healing in ulcer patients.

The implementation of IV therapy for ulcer treatment follows a highly individualized protocol, customized to the unique needs of each patient. Factors influencing the treatment plan include the type and severity of ulcers, nutritional status, and overall health. A potential treatment schedule may involve customized nutrient infusions administered once or twice a month, adjusted based on regular monitoring of nutrient levels and symptom management. Glutamine infusions may be administered once or twice a week for 4-6 weeks, followed by a maintenance schedule tailored to the patient's response to treatment and overall health.

Summary

The burgeoning demand for IV hydration clinics is met with a simultaneous surge in the establishment of such clinics. In order to distinguish oneself in this competitive landscape, it becomes imperative to carve out a niche. Within the pages of this book, we present an extensive overview encompassing vitamins, minerals, amino acids, enzymes, and peptides commonly utilized in IV hydration therapy. While not exhaustive, the compilation is robust, serving as a valuable resource for clinic owners seeking specialization avenues, be it in the realm of IV hydration tailored for specific medical conditions or unique drip formulations.

This comprehensive guide encourages clinic owners to leverage it as foundational knowledge, recognizing that IV hydration formulas are often concocted at the individual clinic level. The absence of a consensus regarding the optimal quantity, frequency, and duration necessitates a thoughtful approach. To assist in this endeavor, we offer solid guidelines that serve as a starting point for meaningful discussions with medical directors and pharmacists to develop customized protocols.

It is crucial to acknowledge the dynamic nature of research in this field, with constant exploration leading to the discovery, promotion, or rediscovery of new elements. To remain at the forefront, it is advised to stay abreast of ongoing research developments for the benefit of both the clinic proprietor and their clientele.

CHAPTER ELEVEN
GUIDELINES

The guidelines outlined in the United States Pharmacopeia (USP) General Chapter 797 serve as a comprehensive framework for the secure compounding of sterile preparations, particularly those intended for intravenous (IV) therapy. This regulatory document has been meticulously developed to mitigate the risk of contamination and uphold the safety and efficacy of compounded sterile preparations, specifically those designed for IV administration. The USP Chapter 797 guidelines encompass a diverse array of facets related to IV therapy, encompassing facilities, equipment specifications, and various procedural considerations.

One crucial aspect delineated in the guidelines pertains to facilities and equipment used in the compounding process. This includes stringent requirements for the design and construction of clean rooms and other compounding areas, as well as detailed specifications for essential equipment such as laminar flow hoods and biological safety cabinets. A clean room or compounding area is a meticulously designated space where sterile preparations are compounded, constructed in adherence to specific design and environmental parameters. These parameters encompass positive air pressure, controlled temperature and humidity levels, adequate air filtration, and circulation. The physical layout ensures the separation of the clean room from other areas within the facility, effectively preventing cross-contamination.

The guidelines further detail the critical role of laminar flow hoods in maintaining a sterile environment during compounding. These hoods employ high-efficiency particulate air (HEPA) filters to purify the incoming air and create a vertical airflow, thereby establishing a sterile work environment. Laminar flow hoods are primarily employed for compounding low and medium-risk sterile preparations. Additionally, the guidelines underscore the significance of biological safety cabinets (BSCs), akin to laminar flow hoods but providing an added layer of protection for both the compounder and the environment. BSCs feature a physical barrier between the compounding area and the operator and utilize HEPA filters for both incoming and outgoing air. These cabinets are specifically designated for compounding high-risk sterile preparations and hazardous drugs.

Equipment and supplies play a pivotal role in sterile compounding, with various items such as vials, syringes, needles, filters, gowns, gloves, and disinfectants being essential components. The guidelines emphasize the imperative that all equipment and supplies utilized in the compounding process must be sterile and non-toxic to ensure the integrity of the preparations. Furthermore, the guidelines introduce the incorporation of environmental monitoring equipment, which is instrumental in assessing the air quality within the compounding area. This equipment measures particle counts, temperature, humidity, and pressure differentials, facilitating ongoing monitoring to guarantee that the compounding area consistently adheres to the required standards for cleanliness and air quality.

Guidelines pertaining to personnel training and qualifications in the context of compounding sterile preparations, particularly intravenous (IV) medications, are detailed below:

a. **Education and Training:**

Personnel engaged in sterile compounding must possess adequate education and training in the compounding of sterile preparations, including IV medications. Additionally, they should demonstrate proficiency in understanding pertinent regulations, standards, and guidelines governing their practice.

b. **Competency Assessment:**

   Ongoing evaluation of personnel's knowledge, skills, and abilities relevant to sterile compounding is imperative. This assessment may involve written and practical tests, along with continuous performance evaluations.

c. **Aseptic Technique:**

   Training in aseptic technique is crucial to prevent the introduction of microorganisms into sterile preparations. This involves comprehensive instruction in proper hand hygiene, gowning, gloving, and disinfection procedures.

d. **Personal Protective Equipment (PPE):**

   Personnel should be well-versed in the correct usage of personal protective equipment, encompassing gowns, gloves, masks, and eye protection. Adequate training should also cover the appropriate disposal procedures for contaminated materials.

e. **Continuing Education:**

   To stay abreast of evolving standards and guidelines in sterile compounding, personnel must engage in continuous education and training.

f. **Supervision:**

   Those involved in sterile compounding should be under the supervision of qualified individuals possessing the requisite knowledge and training in sterile compounding practices.

g. **Classroom Instruction:**

Classroom instruction forms the foundational knowledge base on aseptic technique, sterile compounding, and the compounding process. This may include courses in microbiology, pharmacology, and adherence to standards like USP General Chapter 797.

h. **Hands-on Training:**

Vital for skill development, hands-on training involves instruction on the use of sterile compounding equipment (e.g., laminar flow hoods, syringe pumps) and techniques such as hand hygiene and gowning.

i. **Competency Assessment (Reiteration):**

Reiterating the significance, ongoing competency assessments are integral to ensure personnel possess the necessary knowledge and skills for effective job performance.

j. **Continuing Education (Reiteration):**

Continuous learning is essential to stay current with advancements in aseptic technique, sterile compounding, and the overall compounding process. This includes participating in conferences, workshops, seminars, online courses, and webinars.

k. **Refresher Training:**

Periodic refresher training is vital to reinforce knowledge and skills acquired during initial training, ensuring that personnel consistently demonstrate competence. This may be mandated on an annual or bi-annual basis.

Environmental monitoring plays a crucial role in pharmaceutical and healthcare settings, involving the systematic examination of air and surfaces within clean rooms and compounding areas to ascertain their freedom from contaminants. This comprehensive process encompasses various elements, each contributing to the overall assessment of the environmental conditions in these critical spaces.

a. Particle counts are conducted as part of environmental monitoring, employing a laser particle counter to measure airborne particles in the compounding area. The resulting particle count serves as a metric for evaluating the cleanliness level of the environment and ensuring compliance with established standards.

b. Surface sampling is another integral component of environmental monitoring, involving the collection of samples from surfaces within the compounding area. This is typically achieved using swabs or contact plates. The objective of surface sampling is twofold: to pinpoint potential sources of contamination and to evaluate the efficacy of cleaning procedures implemented in the facility.

c. Microbial testing, a vital aspect of environmental monitoring, may involve analyzing samples for microbial contamination through culture-based or molecular methods. This type of testing is instrumental in identifying potential sources of contamination and assessing the effectiveness of disinfection procedures in place.

d. Monitoring temperature, humidity, and pressure is essential for maintaining a stable and controlled environment conducive to sterile compounding. This is achieved through the use of specialized sensors that measure and record these parameters within the compounding area.

e. Rigorous record-keeping is a fundamental requirement of environmental monitoring. Data collected during monitoring activities should be diligently recorded and maintained for a specified period, in accordance with the facility's policy. Regular review of this data is imperative to identify trends and ensure ongoing compliance with the prescribed standards for the compounding area.

In summary, environmental monitoring encompasses a multifaceted approach to guarantee the cleanliness, sterility, and overall suitability of compounding areas in pharmaceutical and healthcare facilities. The combination of particle counts, surface sampling, microbial testing, environmental parameter monitoring, and robust record-keeping collectively contributes to maintaining high standards in sterile compounding environments.

Cleaning and Disinfection Protocols:

Within the framework of established guidelines, meticulous procedures and specific agents are outlined for the cleaning and disinfection of compounding areas and equipment. These guidelines serve as a comprehensive reference, delineating the requisite steps and materials essential for maintaining a sterile environment.

Compounding Procedures:

The guidelines extend their purview to encompass detailed instructions for the preparation of sterile compounded formulations, with a particular focus on intravenous (IV) medications. Additionally, the guidelines address the handling protocols for hazardous drugs, underscoring the critical importance of adherence to safety measures.

Procedure Execution:

a. Gather Supplies:

Initiate the process by assembling all necessary supplies, including the medication vial, sterile syringe and needle, sterile gloves, alcohol swabs, and a sterile vial adapter.

b. Wash Hands and Don Personal Protective Equipment:

Prioritize hygiene by performing thorough handwashing and donning appropriate personal protective equipment, which includes a sterile gown, gloves, mask, and eye protection.

c. Clean Work Area:

Ensure a pristine work environment by meticulously cleaning the workspace with a disinfectant solution, allowing it to air dry to maintain an aseptic condition.

d. Verify Medication Order:

Conduct a meticulous verification of the medication order against the patient's medical record and the medication label to prevent any potential discrepancies.

e. Prepare the Medication:

Apply aseptic techniques in preparing the medication, incorporating the addition of the necessary diluent to the vial if required. Withdraw the precise amount of medication into the sterile syringe.

f. Attach the Vial Adapter:

Securely attach the sterile vial adapter to the medication vial, ensuring a firm and secure connection.

g. Mix the Medication:

Employ a gentle swirling motion to thoroughly mix the medication, maintaining the integrity of its composition.

h. Attach the Syringe:

Affix the sterile syringe to the vial adapter and meticulously inject the medication into the vial, adhering to precision in the process.

i. Remove the Syringe:

Once the medication transfer is complete, remove the syringe and vial adapter from the vial with utmost care.

j. Label the Syringe:

Accurately label the syringe with the patient's name, medication name and strength, prescribed dose, and expiration date to ensure traceability and patient safety.

k. Clean the Work Area:

Repeat the cleaning process for the work area using a disinfectant solution and allow it to air dry to maintain a sterile environment.

l. Administer the Medication:

Adhere to facility policy while administering the prepared medication via the appropriate IV route, exercising caution and precision.

m. Dispose of Supplies:

Conclude the process by disposing of all used supplies in designated containers, in accordance with established safety and environmental protocols.

Quality control and assurance play a pivotal role in the realm of pharmaceutical compounding, encompassing the rigorous testing of compounded preparations to ascertain their sterility and potency. Additionally, a vigilant monitoring of compounding processes is implemented to promptly identify and rectify any potential issues that may arise during the intricate procedures involved. The guidelines outlined in the United States Pharmacopeia (USP) Chapter 797 are meticulously crafted to uphold the safety and quality standards of intravenous (IV) therapy and other sterile compounding practices.

It is imperative for healthcare providers and facilities to adhere scrupulously to these guidelines, as doing so not only mitigates the risk of adverse events but also ensures favorable patient outcomes. Strict compliance with the stipulated requirements for facilities and equipment is essential to guarantee the safe and effective compounding of sterile preparations, particularly intravenous medications. Regular maintenance and testing of equipment and facilities are indispensable components of the ongoing efforts to align with the rigorous standards articulated in the USP Chapter 797 guidelines.

The USP General Chapter 797 further categorizes Compounded Sterile Preparations (CSPs) into Low-Risk level, which encompasses activities characterized by their minimal complexity and risk. Examples of Low-Risk level CSPs include the simple aseptic transfer of sterile drugs or nutrients into sterile containers, reconstitution of sterile drugs or nutrients using aseptic techniques, and preparation of sterile products employing only sterile ingredients and devices that have undergone terminal sterilization before use.

Moreover, Low-Risk level CSPs extend to the preparation of a single dose of medication for immediate use, reconstitution of a single dose of medication using aseptic techniques, and the preparation of total parenteral nutrition (TPN) solutions utilizing pre-mixed, sterile components. These activities can be carried out either in a cleanroom or in a specifically segregated area that adheres to the prescribed requirements for a low-risk level CSP.

These stringent requirements encompass the application of aseptic techniques and proper hand hygiene, utilization of sterile, single-use devices, regular cleaning and disinfection of the preparation area and equipment, environmental monitoring to ensure air quality and surface cleanliness, and the meticulous labeling of the CSP with information such as the medication name, strength, dose, and beyond-use date. By diligently following these guidelines, healthcare facilities can uphold the highest standards of quality and safety in the compounding of sterile preparations, thereby safeguarding the well-being of patients.

If one harbors an interest in establishing an intravenous (IV) hydration business, a comprehensive understanding of the US Pharmacopeia (USP) General Chapter 797 guidelines is imperative. These guidelines have been meticulously formulated to govern the sterile compounding of IV preparations, with the overarching goal of preventing contamination and upholding the safety and efficacy of compounded sterile preparations, particularly those related to IV medications.

The guidelines encompass a diverse array of facets, ranging from facility design and equipment requisites to personnel training, qualifications, and environmental monitoring. For those embarking on the endeavor of launching an IV hydration business, careful consideration of the following guidelines is paramount:

Facilities and Equipment:

Establishing a dedicated clean room or compounding area specifically designed for the compounding of sterile preparations is essential. This space must adhere to stringent design and environmental specifications, incorporating features such as positive air pressure, controlled temperature and humidity, adequate air filtration, and proper air circulation. Moreover, the compounding area should be physically separated from other sections of the facility to mitigate the risk of cross-contamination. Additionally, the incorporation of laminar flow hoods and biological safety cabinets is indispensable to create and maintain a sterile environment.

Equipment and Supplies:

An array of equipment and supplies is indispensable for sterile compounding, encompassing vials, syringes, needles, filters, gowns, gloves, and disinfectants. It is imperative that all equipment and supplies utilized in the compounding process are sterile and non-toxic.

Personnel Training and Qualifications:

Personnel engaged in sterile compounding must possess relevant education and training in compounding sterile preparations, particularly those associated with IV medications. A comprehensive understanding of pertinent regulations, standards, and guidelines is also imperative. Aseptic technique training, including proper hand hygiene, gowning, gloving, and disinfection procedures, is mandatory. Additionally, personnel should be well-versed in the correct utilization and disposal of personal protective equipment.

Continuing Education:

To ensure ongoing compliance with the latest standards and guidelines for sterile compounding, personnel should partake in continuous education and training. This may involve attending conferences, workshops, seminars, as well as engaging in online courses and webinars. Refresher training is crucial to reinforce initial knowledge and skills, thereby ensuring ongoing competence.

Environmental Monitoring:

Regular monitoring of the air and surfaces within clean rooms and compounding areas is imperative to ascertain their freedom from contaminants. This involves measuring airborne particles, collecting samples from surfaces, and conducting tests for microbial contamination. Monitoring of temperature, humidity, and pressure is also integral.

In conclusion, adherence to the USP General Chapter 797 guidelines is indispensable for the sterile compounding of IV medications to guarantee patient safety and prevent contamination. Those venturing into the ownership of an IV hydration business must diligently follow these guidelines, ensuring that both the facility and personnel are adequately trained and qualified. Furthermore, availing the services of environmental monitoring for IV hydration clinics is advisable, with regular assessments serving as a proactive measure to identify and address potential issues that could compromise patient safety. Consultation with a qualified environmental monitoring service provider is recommended to determine the optimal monitoring schedule in alignment with local regulations and industry best practices.

Made in the USA
Las Vegas, NV
09 December 2024

8ac64474-aba6-4225-a896-1614e13f6e6cR01